Male LUTS/BPH Made Easy

Christopher R. Chapple • Andrea Tubaro
Editors

Male LUTS/BPH Made Easy

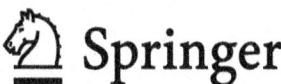 Springer

Editors
Christopher R. Chapple
Department of Urology
Sheffield Teaching Hospitals
NHS Foundation Trust
The Royal Hallamshire Hospital
Sheffield
UK

Andrea Tubaro
Department of Urology
Sant'Andrea Hospital
Rome
Italy

ISBN 978-1-4471-4687-2   ISBN 978-1-4471-4688-9   (eBook)
DOI 10.1007/978-1-4471-4688-9
Springer London Heidelberg New York Dordrecht

© Springer-Verlag London 2014
This work is subject to copyright. All rights are reserved by the Publisher, whether the whole or part of the material is concerned, specifically the rights of translation, reprinting, reuse of illustrations, recitation, broadcasting, reproduction on microfilms or in any other physical way, and transmission or information storage and retrieval, electronic adaptation, computer software, or by similar or dissimilar methodology now known or hereafter developed. Exempted from this legal reservation are brief excerpts in connection with reviews or scholarly analysis or material supplied specifically for the purpose of being entered and executed on a computer system, for exclusive use by the purchaser of the work. Duplication of this publication or parts thereof is permitted only under the provisions of the Copyright Law of the Publisher's location, in its current version, and permission for use must always be obtained from Springer. Permissions for use may be obtained through RightsLink at the Copyright Clearance Center. Violations are liable to prosecution under the respective Copyright Law.
The use of general descriptive names, registered names, trademarks, service marks, etc. in this publication does not imply, even in the absence of a specific statement, that such names are exempt from the relevant protective laws and regulations and therefore free for general use.
While the advice and information in this book are believed to be true and accurate at the date of publication, neither the authors nor the editors nor the publisher can accept any legal responsibility for any errors or omissions that may be made. The publisher makes no warranty, express or implied, with respect to the material contained herein.

Printed on acid-free paper

Springer is part of Springer Science+Business Media (www.springer.com)

We would like to dedicate this work to the many clinical pioneers in the field of functional urology who have led thought and changed our ideas. This work has underpinned all of the information and concepts presented here.

Preface

As men draw near the common goal,
Can anything be sadder,
Than he who, master of his soul,
Is servant to his bladder

–ANONYMOUS

It is a great honour and pleasure to introduce this book on the subject of male LUTS/BPH.

The principle of the book is to emphasise the genesis of thought relating to lower urinary tract symptoms in male patients and to explore the relationship of these symptoms to benign prostatic hyperplasia, emphasising that there are no symptoms pathognomonic of BPH as such. Clearly benign prostatic hyperplasia is a histological condition, which may or may not be associated with symptoms, but which usually results in symptoms as a consequence of obstruction to the bladder outlet (BPO). Having stated this, the book comprehensively reviews the whole subject of LUTS/BPO and the interrelationship with the histological condition BPH.

We believe this book is unique in that it provides a comprehensive and up to date review of this subject in an easily accessible format, as evidenced by the title we have chosen, namely "LUTS/BPO Made Easy". In approximately 160 pages, the whole subject is summarised starting with history and progressing through epidemiology, pathophysiology, clinical assessment, treatment algorithms, medical and various forms of surgical management, leading on to emerging treatments for benign prostatic obstruction and overviewing some of the more challenging clinical issues which may be encountered.

We are particularly proud of the fact that this book has been co-authored with the new generation of young academic urologists.

We hope that you will enjoy this comprehensive and authoritative up-to-date text which truly lives up to the title of "LUTS/BPO Made Easy".

Sheffield, UK
Christopher R. Chapple

Rome, Italy
Andrea Tubaro

Acknowledgements

We would like to thank all of the people who have assisted us in producing this work, in particular Suganya Selvaraj, Andre Tournois and Jen Tidman.

Contents

1 **History of LUTS/BPO and Evolution of Concepts and Terminology**... 1
Roman Sosnowski

2 **Epidemiology and Pathophysiology of LUTS/BPO**................. 21
Alberto Briganti and Giorgio Gandaglia

3 **Assessing LUTS/BPO: What Is the Evidence?**...................... 33
Cosimo De Nunzio and Riccardo Autorino

4 **Treatment Algorithms: When to Treat and Whom?**................ 55
Nikesh Thiruchelvam

5 **Medical Treatment of LUTS/BPH**............................... 67
Giacomo Novara, Vincenzo Ficarra, and Filiberto Zattoni

6 **Open Prostatectomy and Standard Endosurgery**.................. 89
Riccardo Autorino and Cosimo De Nunzio

7 **Surgical Treatment: Lasers and Techniques**...................... 107
Sascha A. Ahyai, Andreas Becker, Malte Rieken, and Alexander Bachmann

8 **Emerging Treatments in BPH**................................... 129
Roman Sosnowski and Nikesh Thiruchelvam

9 **Managing the Complex/Difficult Cases**.......................... 145
Sascha A. Ahyai and Kathrin Simonis

Index... 159

Contributors

Sascha A. Ahyai Department of Urology, University Medical Center Hamburg, Hamburg, Germany

Riccardo Autorino Urology Unit, Second University of Naples, Naples, Italy
YAU-EAU BPH Group, Italy

Alexander Bachmann Department of Urology, University Hospital Basel, Basel, Switzerland

Andreas Becker Department of Urology, University Medical Center Hamburg, Hamburg, Germany

Alberto Briganti Department of Urology, Urological Research Institute, Vita-Salute San Raffaele University, Milan, Italy

Cosimo De Nunzio Department of Urology, Ospedale Sant'Andrea, University "La Sapienza", Rome, Italy
YAU-EAU BPH Group, Rome, Italy

Vincenzo Ficarra Department of Oncological and Surgical Sciences, Urology Clinic, University of Padua, Padua, Italy

Giorgio Gandaglia Department of Urology, Urological Research Institute, Vita-Salute San Raffaele University, Milan, Italy

Giacomo Novara Department of Oncological and Surgical Sciences, Urology Clinic, University of Padua, Padua, Italy

Malte Rieken Department of Urology, University Hospital Basel, Basel, Switzerland

Kathrin Simonis Department of Urology, University Medical Center Hamburg, Hamburg, Germany

Roman Sosnowski Department of Urology, M. Sklodowska-Curie Memorial Cancer Center and Institute of Oncology, Warsaw, Poland

Nikesh Thiruchelvam Department of Urology, Addenbrookes Hospital, Cambridge University Hospitals NHS Trust, Cambridge, UK

Filiberto Zattoni Department of Oncological and Surgical Sciences, Urology Clinic, University of Padua, Padua, Italy

Chapter 1
History of LUTS/BPO and Evolution of Concepts and Terminology

Roman Sosnowski

Abstract The existence of the prostate gland and of prostatic disorders was a mystery for many centuries. Nevertheless, the story of diagnosis and treatment of benign prostatic enlargement (BPE) is one of the most relevant issues in urology and perfectly illustrates the evolution of medicine. The gradual increase of life expectancy over the centuries made possible for chronic disorders associated with aging to develop and for their prevalence to grow. Urinary retention was the most ominous complication of prostatic obstruction leading to renal insufficiency, urinary tract infection, and sometimes death of the patient. Initially, the approach to urinary retention mainly consisted in restoring urethral patency by the means of catheters. Invasive BPH treatments were introduced only in the seventeenth and nineteenth century. Undoubtedly, the technological improvement associated with the industrial revolution resulted in the development of sophisticated devices that could be entered in the male urethra to remove the obstructive adenomatous tissue. The availability of lighting systems and current for electrocautery helped to design the modern electroresectoscope and to develop the technique of transurethral resection of the prostate (TURP). Towards the end of the nineteenth century, surgical techniques for prostate removal were proposed and rapidly developed in the new century. A large number of methods and surgical accesses (retropubic, suprapubic, perineal) prove the complexity of the problem for operators. However, thanks to the evolution of these techniques, adenomectomy has been recognized as the appropriate therapeutic method for "large" prostate adenomas. The technologies available today such as laparoscopy or surgical robots "imitate" the principles of adenomectomy developed many years ago.

The pathophysiology of benign prostatic enlargement remains an elusive issue beyond the obvious permissive role of androgens. Lower urinary tract symptoms, once uniquely associated with BPE in the male patient, now recognize different

R. Sosnowski
Department of Urology, M. Sklodowska-Curie Memorial Cancer Center, and Institute of Oncology, Roentgena 5, Warsaw 02-781, Poland
e-mail: roman.sosnowski@gmail.com

underlying disorders involving the central and peripheral nervous system, the urinary bladder, the prostate, and the pelvic floor. A consensus as to the terminology of LUTS and prostate disorders has been achieved although proper terminology is not always implemented. The diagnosis and management of benign prostatic enlargement and LUTS remains a challenge for the practicing urologist.

Keywords Prostate • Benign prostatic hyperplasia • BPH • Benign prostatic obstruction • BPO • TURP • Adenomectomy • Perineal prostatectomy • Suprapubic prostatectomy • Prostatism • Lower urinary tract symptoms • LUTS • History of urology

Prostate

Micturition disorders have been a challenge in medicine throughout history. Even though at the time of the Roman Empire, the average man's life expectancy was 30 years, while at the end of the nineteenth century, it was 50; the help for prostate sufferers was unsatisfactory and burdened with manifold complications. On the one hand, the history of treating benign prostatic enlargement is a beautiful example on how a scientific and technical thought "pushed" the development of medicine from simple treatments through extensive operations to minimally invasive techniques, and on the other hand, how difficult and burdened with many sorrows the process was.

The word prostate, which means "one who stands before," is derived from the Greek προ, "before," and χισταναι, "to stand" [1]. In ancient Greek, the masculine term prostatēs meant "president" and was exclusively used in a nonmedical sense.

Benign Prostatic Hyperplasia

For many centuries, a reason for urination problems had been unknown and even was to little information of prostate as an organ. Herophilus (first half of the third century BC) and Galen (129–199) the great anatomists probably could recognize the prostate as a separate organ [2]. For many centuries, urinary calculi were regarded as the cause of the urination problems, without noticing the presence of prostate in human anatomy. Leonardo da Vinci (1452–1519) who created impressive anatomical and medical artworks, like his contemporaries, did not notice the presence of prostate as most of his knowledge derived from anatomical dissections of castrated oxen merely having a tiny and atrophic prostate. The "Anatomiae Liber Introductorius" made by Nicola Massa (1504–1589) in 1536 and the "Tabulae Anatomicae" created by the anatomist Andreas Vesalius (1514–1564) in 1538 both displayed the prostate gland for the first time (Fig. 1.1). Vesalius depicted "corpus glandulosum as a single structure" and did more detailed presentation which can be found in "de Humani corporis fabrica Libri septem" from 1543 [3].

1 History of LUTS/BPO and Evolution of Concepts and Terminology

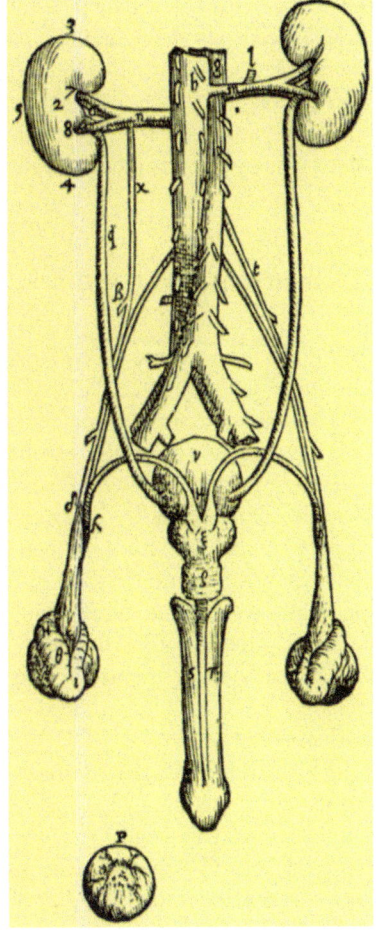

Fig. 1.1 Anterior view of the male genitalia, Andreas Fabrica Vesalius book V: 1543, figure XXIII, p 374. Description: *a* bladder, *b* vesiculae seminales, *c* prostate (*Source*: Mattelaer and Schultheiss [1])

In 1651, Nathaniel Highmore, English surgeon and anatomist (1613–1685), uses a referent "prostate," and in 1792, William Cheselden (1688–1752) postulated that "Prostata are two glands or rather one with the size of a nutney." In 1649, Jean Riolan (1577–1657) was seemingly the first to propose that "the enlarged prostate could cause urinary retention" [4]. He insisted that the neck of the bladder may be closed by "a tumour of the prostate gland." Much emphasis was laid on inflammation as a cause of the prostatic enlargement, gonorrhea being singled out as a particularly important factor. This belief led to a faulty association between venereal diseases and prostatic hyperplasia, which persisted for a long time.

In 1841, Louis Auguste Mercier (1811–1882) was the first to apply the term "hypertrophy" in his work "Recherches Sur Le Traitement Des Maladies Des Organs Urinaires" [5]. Oswald Lowsley (1884–1955) who examined the anatomy of the human prostate did the first anatomical characterization in 1912 – the prostate was "histologically homogenous" and composed of "five discrete lobes" [6]. In

1953, Salvador Gil Vernet (1893–1987) showed in his book that the prostate gland is heterogeneous and build up of two main parts: "the cranial and the caudal gland." Later, Mc Neal affirmed Gil Vernet's findings and reported a "central zone," a "peripheral zone," and a "transition zone" based on three determining factors: histological variety, ductile topography, and the spatial relation to the urethra and ejaculatory ducts [7]. His theoretical account evolved over 20 years [8, 9].

Transurethral Procedures

Although the problem of emptying the urinary bladder was observed for many centuries, the only effective way to help the sufferers was to introduce a tube into it. Thus, Hippocrates advocated that acute retention ought to be cured by purging. The development of the urinary metal catheter is credited to the Romans (Fig. 1.2), Celsus and Galen in the first century AD, and the earliest known description of a flexible catheter was by Avicenna of Arabia in 1036. Catheters were made of a variety of materials from the hollow leaves (e.g., allium fistulosum employed by the ancient Chinese), bamboo, wood, and metal along with rubber and gum, elastic substances of our times, and have been a fundamental method for treating prostatic blockade for 100 years [10]. Patients with recurrent urinary retention had to catheterize themselves repeatedly and constantly carry a catheter in a pocket case, a walking stick, or a designed elaborate cabinet for the use by the patient (Fig. 1.3).

Along with a catheter, various treatments and techniques were tried to alleviate prostatic obstruction. In 1575, Ambroise Pare (1510–1590) presented an innovative surgical procedure using a sound with sharp ridges, approximately a finger's breadth from the apex to extract occluding tissue at the bladder neck [11]. His experiments were far ahead of those made by his contemporaries.

Jean Civiale (1796–1867) from Paris devised the "kiotome" around 1830 for an incision of the obstructing bladder neck. In 1836, his contemporary Louis Auguste Mercier (1811–1882) introduced an instrument called "prostatome" used to incise the median bar or even to remove small tissue particles similar to a prostatic punch. Mercier used this tool about 300 times and thought well of it, but it caused considerable hemorrhage and most patients were left with urinary incontinence. Among many other concepts (various prostate snares, excisors, and incisors) constructed among others by Frenchmen d'Etoilles, Englishman Guthrie, and others, the Mercier's instrument offered the advantage of actually removing the prostate or bladder neck. These blind techniques often caused dramatic hemorrhage and were largely abandoned.

In 1874, Enrico Bottini (1835–1903) from Pavia in Italy was the first to make the transition to electric prostatic surgery. He developed "cauterio termogalvanico" which facilitated destruction and incision of the prostate lobe and median bar without causing a hemorrhage. The procedure was blind and later it was improved by A. Freudenberg who incorporated a telescope (1897) and a more efficient cooling

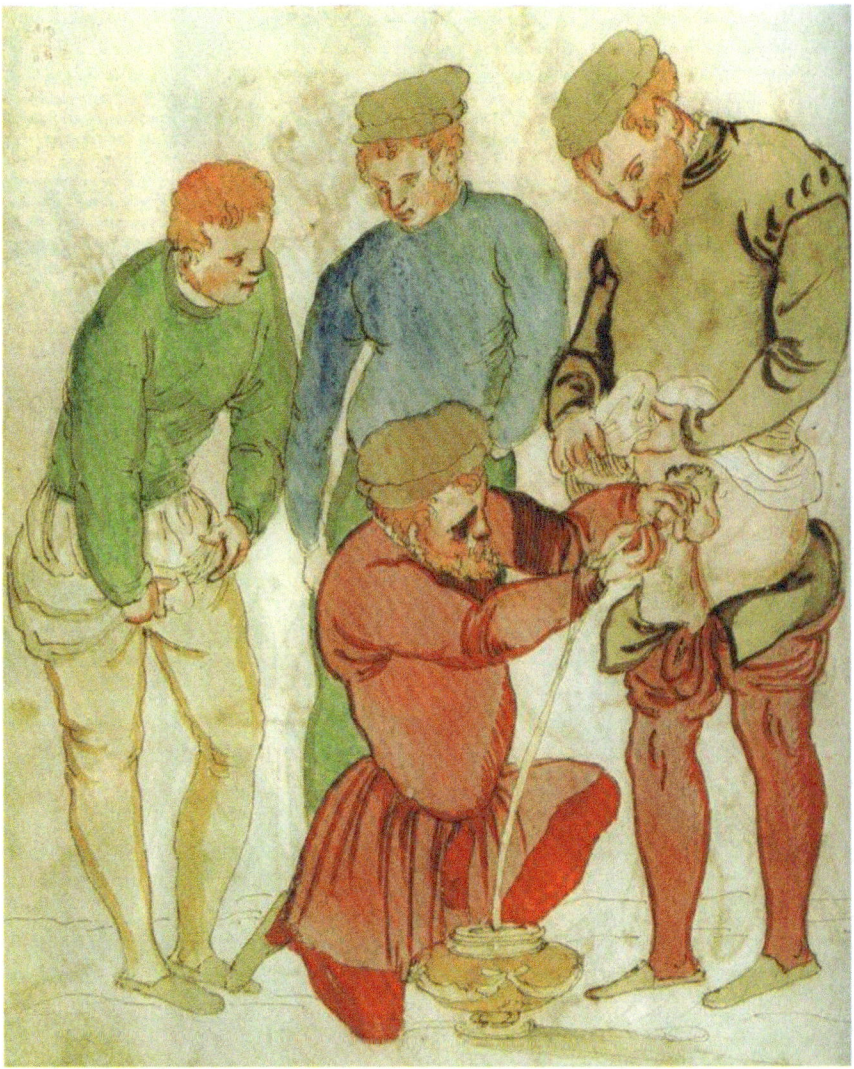

Fig. 1.2 Catheterisation in standing position: Wundarzt in kurzer Robe setzt einem Patienten einen Katheter, illustration by Heinrich Kullmauer and Albrecht Meher from a sketchbook, drawing with watercolours, British Museum, London (*Source*: Mattelaer and Schultheiss [1])

system. As a result, the procedure could be performed under direct vision, but it was still suitable only for smaller prostates and median bars. In 1909, Hugh H. Young (1870–1945) showed his transurethral prostatic punch, which offered an alternative to galvanocautery; however, the cutting procedure was blind and the incidence of hemorrhage correspondingly high (Fig. 1.4).

Lack of vision was a major problem in all these instruments, so quickly they paved the way for cutting-loop resectoscopes.

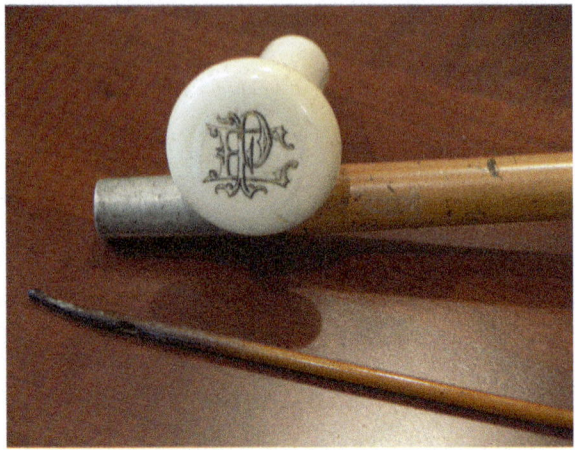

Fig. 1.3 Stashed discreetly in hollow cane-shafts or hatbands, catheters were used to relieve bladder outlet obstruction at the end of the nineteenth century (Image courtesy of the William P. Didusch Museum of the American Urological Association)

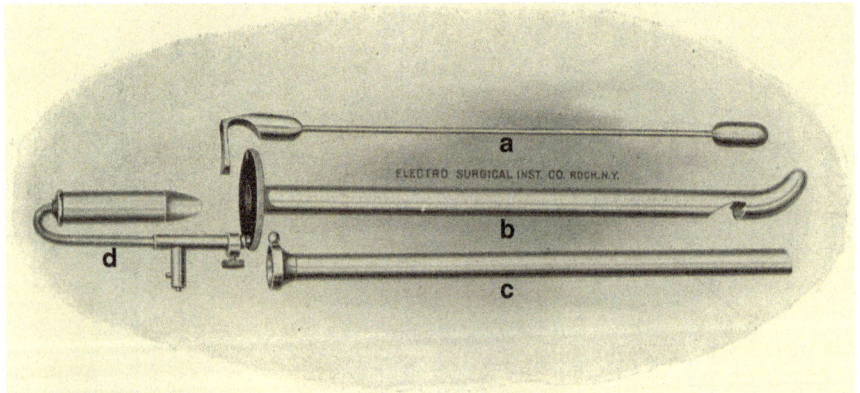

Fig. 1.4 The urethroscopic median bar excisor or punch devised by Hugh Hampton Young in 1901. (**a**) Obturator. (**b**) Outer tube with fenestra to entrap median bar. (**c**) Cutting inner tube. (**d**) Light carrier (*Source*: Mattelaer and Schultheiss [1])

Thanks to the invention of German physician Maximilian Nitze (1848–1906) who in 1877 designed the first successful modern cystoscope, it was possible to improve visualization during intraurethral procedures. Introducing by Josef Leiter (1830–1890) of Vienna incandescent lighting provided by an electrically heated platinum wire that required adding a cooling system of flowing ice water and telescopic lenses for visualization solved many of the problems with earlier instruments. Also, the discovery of high-frequency current by Heinrich Hertz allowed urologists to turn their attention to the least invasive approach to the prostate.

In 1910, Edwin Beer (1876–1938) announced his successful use of high-frequency unipolar current (Oudin) in the treatment of bladder tumors. Beer's outstanding finding was that he discovered a way to cauterize tissue through a cystoscope underwater [12]. These high-frequency currents did not penetrate and damage the surrounding tissue as much as cautery heat, so they produced less necrotic tissue and were less likely to cause secondary hemorrhage. Resection of the prostate with high-frequency current was performed for the first time in 1926 by C.W. Collings from New York. For this purpose, he used a tube machine, which he called a "radiotherm." When he replaced the tube with a high-frequency spark gap, he found that the cutting power did not diminish but there was very little coagulation.

The most important development took place in 1926 when Maximilian Stern (1873–1946) from New York invented a cutting loop of tungsten enabling to pass current, in effect coagulating while cutting [13]. He described an instrument capable of operating in water medium, capable of extracting a longitudinal "spaghetti-like" segment of tissue; he named this tool a "resectoscope." His first report compromised 46 patients with no bleeding or other unfavorable reaction.

In 1931, Theodore M. Davis (1889–1937), who had been an electrical engineer before entering the field of urology, combined the cutting current with a diathermy machine for hemostasis and reported good results. Davis improved the loops by using larger tungsten wire cutting loop on Stern's resectoscope, which made it stronger and less prone to breakage. He provided better insulation, which was badly needed. Later, with Bovie, he constructed "Davies–Bovie Electrocautery Equipment" containing first dual-action foot switch, allowing direct control of either cutting or coagulating current, which is still in use today (Fig. 1.5).

Inspired by Davis, Joseph F. McCarthy (1877–1946) from New York made significant improvements in a resectoscope. One of McCarthy's major inventions was the attachment of an insulating Bakelite resectoscope sheath, which enabled direct visualization and precise control of the movements of the cutting loop in a safe manner, even while current was used, posing no electrical risk to the operator [14]. However, the key to the success of this instrument was a wonderful foroblique telescope developed by Reinhold Wappler. It provided both a wide-angle view and sufficient magnification allowing the precise placement and manipulation of the cutting loop. The Stern–McCarthy resectoscope, as it is currently known, was the first practical cutting-loop resectoscope and marks the beginning of the modern era of transurethral prostate surgery (Fig. 1.6). When first introduced, standard transurethral prostate resection with the Stern–McCarthy instrument involved removal of only a few segments from an obstructing median bar or the lateral lobe. A typical operative report of the era would state "adequate channel made," "5 pieces burned out," or "3 segments of prostate removed." Mortality rates from early transurethral prostate surgeries were as high as 25 %. In 1939, Reed Nesbitt designed a spring trigger allowing one-handed resection. A benefit of this method was that the prostate could be elevated rectally with the free hand, providing more of a depth impression during the procedure of prostatectomy [15]. Transurethral resection of the prostate emerged as a dominant method for the treatment of the enlarged prostate and this technique was used extensively in the following years.

In 1932, Joseph F. McCarthy introduced the first modern resectoscope with a 2-handed rack-and-pinion-style working element and improved Stern-type tungsten wire cutting loop, Davis' dual-control foot switch, the Wappler foroblique

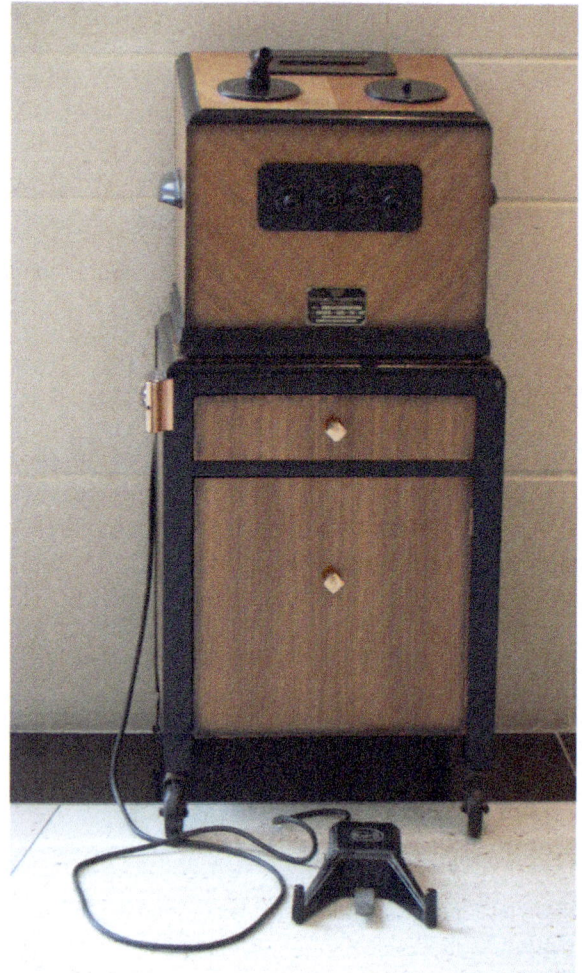

Fig. 1.5 Davis-Bovie generator of the 1930s (Image courtesy of the William P. Didusch Museum of the American Urological Association)

direct-vision telescope, and Wappler electrical unit with both dampened spark-gap coagulating and vacuum tube-based cutting currents.

Transurethral prostatectomy, as we know it today, could not have been developed without four landmark inventions: a cystoscope, the first practical incandescent light bulb, the fenestrated tube, and the application of high-frequency electrical current underwater [1]. In the second half of the twentieth century, further improvements were created, including the invention of the rod-lens system [16].

Another novelty involved a change of irrigation fluid from water to glycine [17]. The most recent major improvement is the introduction of microchip cameras in the last decade, and since then, TURP has become much easier to teach and assess. Consequently, TURP has evolved into one of the safest, most effective, and widely used procedures for the extirpation of the hyperplasic prostate.

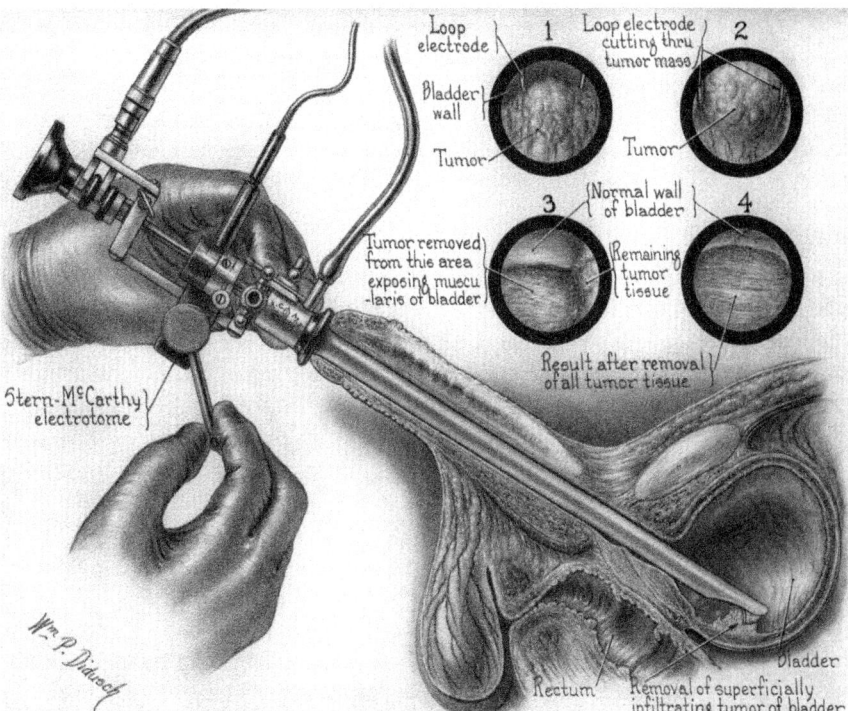

Fig. 1.6 The Stern-McCarthy prostatic resectoscope (*Source*: Image courtesy of the William P. Didusch Museum of the American Urological Association)

Operative Procedures

During the second half of the nineteenth century, perineal prostatectomy developed along with two parallel paths. Suprapubic removal of the prostate was first carried out in 1885, and it was followed by uncountable endoscopic incisions, forages, and cauterizations, the endoscopic punch procedure, and later endoscopic resection of the prostate.

Perineal Prostatectomy

The first perineal access was described for lithotomy. Later, several attempts were made to apply the same access in perineal prostatectomy. Partial prostatectomies have undoubtedly been performed accidentally during perineal lithotomy. According to Bryant's recommendation in elderly patients during lithotomy, all the prostate tissue has to be extracted to resolve the symptoms of obstructive micturition [1].

George Goodfellow (1855–1910) performed the first perineal enucleation of the enlarged prostate in 1891. In 1904, he gave the first account on 72 cases which "he had operated with only 2 fatalities" [18]. Many surgeons followed him and contributed various technical aspects to perineal prostatectomy. The visualized extraurethral technique used today was developed almost simultaneously by Zuckerkandl (1899), Proust [19], and Hugh Young [20]. It was associated with the developments in the form of appropriate perineal retractors, along with an exaggerated dorsal lithotomy position [19, 20]. Postoperative complications such as rectourethral fistula, urinary incontinence, and particularly impotence caused that in Europe such operations were avoided contrary to America, where the enthusiasm, better anatomical knowledge, and persistence of Hugh Young, together with his growing reputation, allowed the technique to flourish. It became arguably a more widespread technique than suprapubic prostatectomy within the USA during the early twentieth century. Later, Young described the technique on malignant (1905) prostates.

Suprapubic Prostatectomy

The fear, which originated in the Hippocratic belief that bladder wounds were fatal, retarded the development of suprapubic prostatectomy. The first suprapubic access to the bladder was made by Nicholas Franco of Lausanne (1556) for stone extraction, but this was only done in desperation after the failure of the perineal technique. The earliest record of suprapubic prostatectomy is dated on 1827 when Jean Amussat (1796–1856) used scissors to cut away the obstructing prominent middle lobe. During the late nineteenth century, various surgeons, including Billroth, von Dittel, and Trendelenburg, described numerous techniques of suprapubic prostatectomy, but it was not performed frequently until the end of the century. William Belfield analyzed all the published cases of prostatectomy in 1890. He found 133 operations, including 88 suprapubic, and the rest being perineal or combinations of techniques [21]. Along with Arthur McGill, they were the first real advocates of suprapubic prostatectomy [22] and the first to report series complications of the operations. In 1892, the mortality of suprapubic prostatectomy was >20 %.

It seems likely that the first operations before 1895 were only partial prostatectomies. A credit for the first deliberate suprapubic enucleation of the whole prostate gland goes to Eugene Fuller from New York. He published an account of six cases of "prostatectomy" he had done by the suprapubic route and drained through the perineum. Realizing that unfavorable results of other operators who merely aimed to chisel out a channel were caused by incomplete excision of the enlarged gland, Fuller first cut the bladder neck with scissors to localize the plane between the adenoma and capsule and then used his finger to remove both lateral and median lobes [23]. Sir Peter Freyer, in a paper "Total Extirpation of the Prostate for Radical Cure of Enlargement of that Organ," claimed to have performed the first complete enucleation of the prostate by the suprapubic route. He described a method much alike to Fuller's, apart from the fact that he scored the urothelium with his fingernail rather than scissors and inserted a considerable suprapubic drain without urinary catheter [24, 25].

In its original form, the Fuller–Freyer prostatectomy was a relatively unsophisticated operation performed in two steps: at first, enucleation, followed by compressive hemostasis and cystostomy. Some weeks later, cystostomy was closed. Although undoubtedly Fuller was an originator of the operation, Freyer was the first to show it could be done safely and expeditiously, this being particularly important before the sophisticated anesthetic agents and muscle relaxants appeared. In suprapubic prostatectomies performed in 1625, he reported a mortality rate of 5.3 %, which is very favorable with "catheter life" in the early twentieth century having 8 % mortality in the first month of application [26].

As the surgical methods developed, operators turned to reducing morbidity, especially, by hemostasis. E.L. Keynes from America presented numerous hemostatic techniques such as cautery, stitches, tamponade, and pressure [27]. Hugh Young developed his "boomerang" needle to lay sutures deep in the prostatic fossa and Paul Pilcher described a hemostatic bag. All these techniques were to some extent successful.

Another variant of suprapubic prostatectomy, created by Harry Harris in the late 1920s, was the next breakthrough in this field [28]. By seaming the trigone muscle to the floor of the prostatic cavity and then shutting the cavity by suturing it around an indwelling catheter, Harris obtained a primary closure of the bladder [29]. This method was later ameliorated by Hryntschack [30].

Retropubic Prostatectomy

"Prostatectomia suprapubica extravesicalis" had already been performed by W.J. van Stockum (1860–1913) in 1908 who did not open the bladder but simply incised the capsule of the prostate to shell out the adenoma. He packed the cavity with gauze and drained the bladder with a suprapubic tube.

However, the wide clinical establishment of retropubic approach to the prostatic gland after 1945 must be attributed to the Irish surgeon Terence J. Millin (1903–1980), who worked in London [31]. This procedure gave several benefits to the patient: an intact bladder and effective closure and scabbing of the prostatic capsule, along with a shorter and more convenient convalescence [1]. The Millin's technique was quickly adopted as the operation of choice within the UK and revolutionized urological practice worldwide (Fig. 1.7).

Conservative Treatment

The turn of the century marked a growing interest in orchidectomy as a treatment for the enlarged prostate although then the particular association with prostate cancer was not known. William White noticed that the symptoms improved in over a

RETROPUBIC URINARY SURGERY

BY

TERENCE MILLIN

M.A., M.Ch. (Dubl.), F.R.C.S., F.R.C.S.I.

Surgeon, All Saints' Hospital for Genito-Urinary Diseases, London; Genito-Urinary Surgeon, Royal Masonic Hospital, London; Urologist, Surrey County Council; Genito-Urinary Surgeon, Chelsea Hospital for Women, London; Southall-Norwood and Cray Valley Hospitals.

BALTIMORE
THE WILLIAMS AND WILKINS COMPANY
1947

Fig. 1.7 (**a**) Front page of the Millin's book "Retropubic Urinary Surgery" 1947, Livingstone LTD (*Source*: Image courtesy of the William P. Didusch Museum of the American Urological Association). (**b**) Millin's technic of retropubic prostatectomy (*Source*: Image courtesy of the William P. Didusch Museum of the American Urological Association)

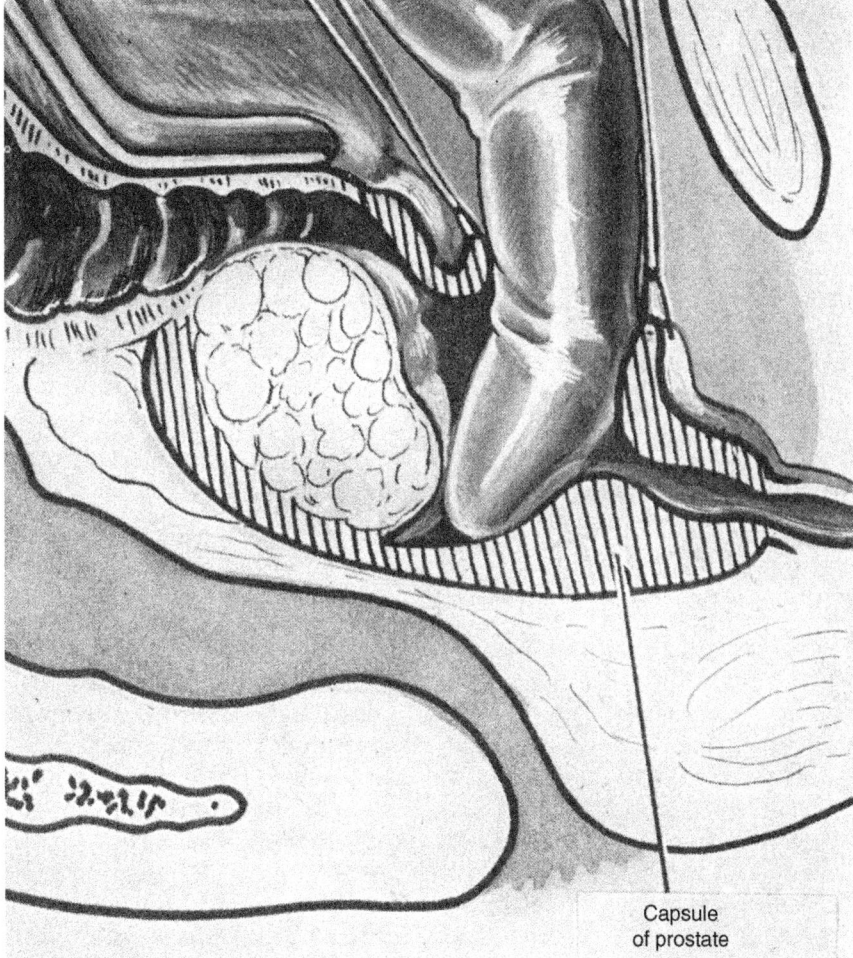

Fig. 1.7 (continued)

half of patients with an enlarged prostate treated by castration [32]. However, despite these seminal works, orchidectomy never found favor with practitioners of the day. In 1893, August Bier ligated both internal iliac arteries in the hope of causing ischemic atrophy of the prostate, but in his series of 11 patients, three died. Other surgical methods were tested, including vasectomy, with little success [33].

Present and Future Concepts of Treatment

The process of understanding the pathogenesis of benign prostatic enlargement, the lower urinary tract symptoms, and the methods of their treatment is a good example of changes that occur in medicine, in this case in urology, starting from a simple introduction of a catheter through open operations to minimally invasive techniques – this is the history of treating BPE. Nowadays, less invasive therapeutic techniques are available. Patients and doctors' choice is dictated by a desire to achieve the best possible quality of life after the treatment. Our offer includes, among others, TUNA (transurethral needle ablation), TUMT (transurethral microwave thermotherapy), TULIP (transurethral ultrasound-guided laser-induced prostatectomy), TUIP (transurethral incision of the prostate), TUVP (transurethral electrovaporization of the prostate), TUEP (transurethral evaporation of the prostate), HoLEP (holmium laser enucleation of the prostate), PVP (photo vaporization of the prostate), LSP (laparoscopic simple prostatectomy), RASP (robotic-assisted simple prostatectomy), and R-STEP (robotic single port suprapubic transvesical enucleation of the prostate).

Evolution of Concepts and Terminology of LUTS/BPO

Prostatism

Historically, many terms have been used to describe the urinary symptoms in men. Due to the location of the prostate and its spatial relation to the urethra and bladder, this organ and its pathology was regarded a fundamental cause of the symptoms mentioned above. The term "prostatism" was used to describe any urination-related symptoms caused by the pathology of this organ.

The term "prostatism" has been coined partly as a result of the commercial interest, patients' rising awareness and demands, and partly by the advent of new treatments [34]. The actions of pharmaceutical companies had a significant impact on the use of this term, as they put a lot of effort into increasing the awareness of prostatic disease both in patients and doctors. The term "prostatism" was used only in men in connection with "symptoms of benign prostatic enlargement." Initially, the two groups of symptoms were assigned to the term "prostatism": "irritative" and "obstructive." Additionally, the term "irritative" was associated with the symptoms of urinary infection or inflammation.

Lower Urinary Tract Symptoms

In the 90s, it was noticed that the similar urinary symptoms occurred in women; therefore, the use of the term "prostatism" was no longer justified. In summary of his work, Paul Abrams found that no symptoms are typical of either benign prostatic enlargement or one of its consequences – bladder outflow obstruction [35]. In addition, he noticed that BPH is a histological definition, according to which the condition occurs in 88 % of men over the age of 80 years. He also added that if some men demonstrate the prostate enlargement, it should be defined as "benign prostatic enlargement" (BPE) [34]. According to Abrams, half of men with BPE develop "true bladder outlet obstruction" and this state should be defined as "benign prostatic obstruction" (BPO). Already in 1984, Barry reported that histological BPH was not observed in men under the age of 30; however, its incidence rose with age, topping out a maximum in the ninth decade [36]. In the previously cited study, Abrams concluded that the use of the term "prostatism" is not justified for several reasons. Firstly, the expressions such as prostatism and clinical benign prostatic hyperplasia imply sham diagnostic authority, which may be interpreted as therapy without proper diagnosis. Secondly, approximately one third of men with prostatism do not demonstrate bladder outflow obstruction as a consequence of the prostatic enlargement. A lot of men with prostatism and without bladder outflow obstruction have an unsatisfactory result of prostatectomy. In addition, transurethral resection of the prostate is connected with low but meaningful morbidity and mortality: Death of some men may be needless [34]. The author proposed the introduction of the term "lower urinary tract symptoms" (LUTS), which describes patients' ailments without implying their cause and that is suitable to any patient with urinary symptoms, regardless of age and sex [34]. Furthermore, taking into account the pathophysiology of these symptoms, he suggested replacing the currently used terms with the new ones. Thus, "storage symptoms" would be more suitable than "irritative symptoms" (frequent urination, urgency, and urgent incontinence in most cases suggest a functional abnormality) and "voiding symptoms" could substitute the expression "obstructive symptoms" (hesitancy, poor flow of urine, straining, urinary retention, and intermittency) [34]. In subsequent years, international scientific conferences devoted to this issue confirmed a legitimacy of using the term LUTS. In 1997, the 4th International Consultation on BPH decided that the expression LUTS should replace "prostatism," as a cause-and-effect BPH-symptom relationship has not been demonstrated [37].

In 2000, the 5th International Consultation on Benign Prostatic Hyperplasia, which took place in Paris, found the term LUTS justified, as it refers broadly to various combinations of both irritative and obstructive or filling and voiding symptoms, which are so frequent in aging men. Secondly, the expression does not allege to create a cause-and-effect relationship between the symptoms and any specific organ, i.e., prostate, bladder neck, bladder, or urethra [38]. It has been assumed that the term LUTS describes a combination of symptoms such as irritative and/or obstructive voiding disturbances, which are frequent in aging men. This can be accompanied by enlarged prostate gland (EPG), bladder outlet obstruction (BOO) (suspected or urodynamically confirmed), and stromo-glandular hyperplasia of the prostatic gland called benign prostatic hyperplasia (BPH). However, the association of any of these conditions does not necessarily suggest a causal relationship, though the enlarged prostate may be responsible for LUTS [38]. Finally, lower urinary tract symptoms have been specified by the standardization subcommittee of the International Continence Society (ICS) in February 2002: "LUTS are the subjective indicators of a disease or change in conditions as perceived by the patients, carer or partners and may lead him/her to seek help from health care professionals.

Symptoms may either be volunteered or described during the patient interview. They are usually qualitative" [39]. LUTS was divided into three groups: "filling/storage symptoms" (frequent urination, nocturia, compelling urge to urinate, urinary incontinence, stress or urge incontinence, inability to control urination, nocturnal enuresis, continuous loss of bladder control, bladder sensation), "emptying/voiding symptoms" (slow flow of urine, splitting, irregularity of voiding, hesitancy, pressing to void, final dribbling), and "post-micturition symptoms" (urinary retention, post-micturition dribbling) [39].

Popularization of the term LUTS in the twenty-first century and the attempts to explain the pathophysiology of this problem resolved inaccuracies in terminology and the misleading meaning of the previous application of the "BPH" phrase. The following terms associated with the lower urinary tract pathology have been introduced: BPH, benign prostatic hyperplasia (characteristic histopathological model); BPE, benign prostatic enlargement (benign enlargement caused by a nonmalignant lesion); BPO, benign prostatic obstruction (bladder outlet obstruction); DO, detrusor overactivity; and OAB, overactive bladder, regarded crucial to describe clinical findings [40]. Mutual relations between these concepts were most often presented in the form of diagrams. They displayed overlapping circles that symbolized the situations where one patient developed one, two, or more clinical conditions simultaneously.

In 2006, Chapple and Roehrborn emphasised that the presence of LUTS does not need to be associated with the prostatic pathology only. In their study, the authors recommend correct terminology [41]. Thus, the term benign prostatic enlargement (BPE) ought to be applied when BPH has not been histologically proven. BPE may be a reason for bladder outlet obstruction (BOO), which is manifested as increased detrusor pressure and decreased urine flow rate. Moreover, a diagnosis of BOO is made using simultaneous measuring of flow rate and detrusor pressure determined in the urodynamic pressure–flow tests. They measure both static (elevated tissue mass) and dynamic (raised smooth muscle tonus) constituent of the prostate. LUTS should be applied until pressure–flow tests have proven BOO, as many men with LUTS do not manifest BOO. In summary, the authors conclude that "LUTS may result from a complex interplay of pathophysiological influences, including prostatic pathology and bladder dysfunction" [41]. The term covers all storage and voiding symptoms. The expression LUTS should be used instead of BPH or BOO until the latter is diagnosed using adequate examinations. Even though the enlarged prostatic gland can be responsible for the onset of LUTS in men over the age of 40, other causes are of equal significance. The most recent reports suggest that LUTS may be connected with the prostate (BPH–LUTS), bladder (detrusor overactivity–overactive bladder syndrome [OAB], detrusor underactivity), or kidney (increased nocturnal urine output) [41]. Inappropriate use of terminology can lead to misunderstandings between doctors and patients resulting in mismanagement of the conditions that underlie LUTS in men.

A variety of LUTS causes have been illustrated in Fig. 1.8. It is believed that a single person complaining of LUTS has more than one of these factors. This multifactorial view on the LUTS etiology has led most specialists to consider the whole urinary system as a single functional item [42].

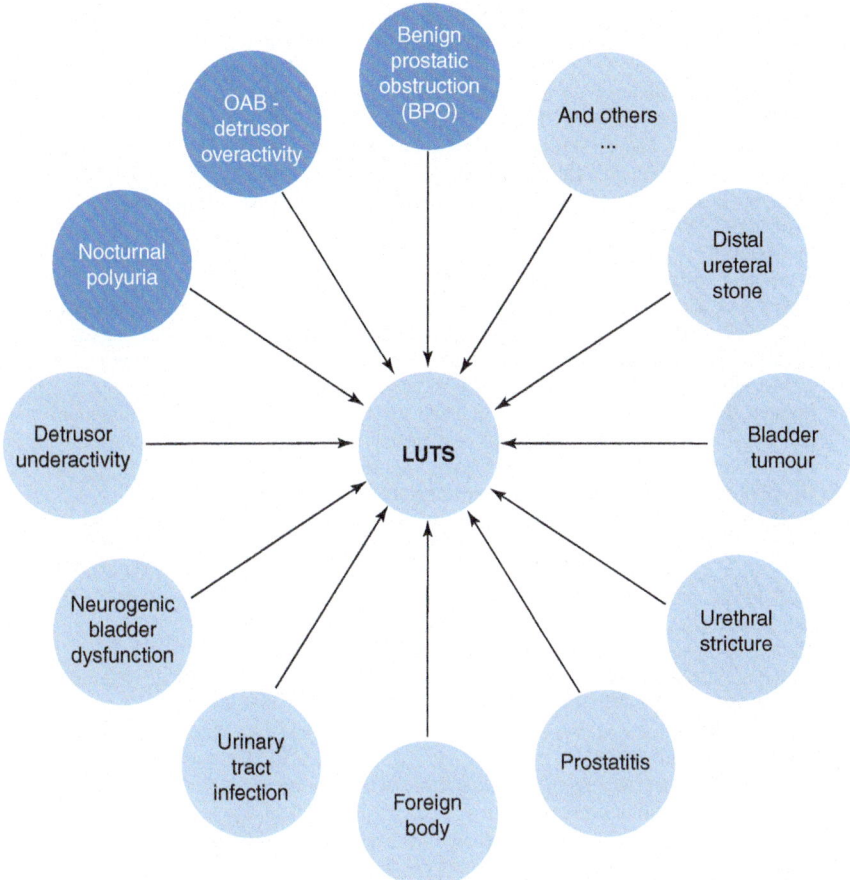

Fig. 1.8 Multifactorial aetiology of lower urinary tract symptoms (LUTS) (*Source*: Oelke et al. [42])

References

1. Mattelaer J, Schultheiss D. Europe – the cradle of urology. Arnhem: History Office of the European Association of Urology; 2010. p. 164–72.
2. Shelley HS. The enlarged prostate: a brief history of its treatment. J Hist Med Allied Sci. 1969;24:452–73.
3. Marx FJ, Karenberg A. History of the term prostate. Prostate. 2009;69(2):208–13. PubMed PMID: WOS:000262701200011. English.
4. Herr HW. The enlarged prostate: a brief history of its surgical treatment. BJU Int. 2006;98(5):947–52. PubMed PMID: 17034596.
5. Mercier LA. Recherches sur le traitement des maladies organes urinaires. 1856; 36–213.
6. Oswald LS. The development of the human prostate gland with reference to the development of other structures at the neck of the bladder. Am J Anat. 1912;131:299–349.
7. Selman SH. The McNeal prostate: a review. Urology. 2011;78(6):1224–8. PubMed PMID: 21908026.
8. McNeal JE. Regional morphology and pathology of the prostate. Am J Clin Pathol. 1968;49(3):347–57.

9. McNeal JE. Normal histology of the prostate. Am J Surg Pathol. 1988;12(8):619–33.
10. Shackley D. A century of prostatic surgery. BJU Int. 1999;83(7):776–82. PubMed PMID: 10368195. English.
11. Rognon LM, Raymond G. A historical overview of benign prostatic hyperplasia. Ann Urol. 1992;26(3):167–87. PubMed PMID: WOS:A1992JG53200007. French.
12. Beer E. Removal of neoplasms of the urinary bladder; a new method, employing high-frequency (oudin) currents through a catheterizing cystoscope. Am J Med. 1910;54(22):1768–9.
13. Stern M. Resection of obstruction at the vesical orifice; new instruments and new method. JAMA. 1926;87(21):1726–30.
14. McCarthy JF. A new apparatus for endoscopic plastic surgery of the prostate, diathermia and excision of vesical growths. J Urol. 1931;26:695–9.
15. Nesbit RM. Modification of the Stern-McCarthy resectoscope permitting 3D perception during transurethral prostatectomy. J Urol. 1939;41:646–8.
16. Hopkins HH, Kapany NS. A flexible fibrescope, using static scanning. Nature. 1954;173((4392):39–41. PubMed PMID: WOS:A1954UA36600025. English.
17. Emmett JL, Gilbaugh Jr JH, McLean P. Fluid absorption during transurethral resection: comparison of mortality and morbidity after irrigation with water and non-hemolytic solutions. J Urol. 1969;101(6):884–9. PubMed PMID: 5771262.
18. Goodfellow G. Median perineal prostatectomy. JAMA. 1904;7:194–7.
19. Proust R. Technique de la prostatectomie périnéale. Ass Franc Urol. 1901;5:361–74.
20. Young HH. Conservative perineal prostatectomy; a presentation of new instruments and technic. JAMA. 1903;10:999–1009.
21. Belfield WI. Operation on the enlarged prostate, with a tabulated summary of cases. M J Med Sci. 1890;100:439–52.
22. McGill AF. Suprapubic prostatectomy. Br Med J. 1887;2:1104–5.
23. Fuller E. Six successful and successive cases of prostatectomy. J Cutan Genitourin Dis. 1895;6:229–39.
24. Freyer PJ. A new method of performing perineal prostatectomy. Br Med J. 1900;1(2047):698–9. PubMed PMID: 20758920. Pubmed Central PMCID: 2505977.
25. Freyer PJ. A clinical lecture on total extirpation of the prostate for radical cure of enlargement of that organ: with four successful cases. Br Med J. 1901;2:125–8.
26. Blandy JP. Surgery of the benign prostate. First Sir Peter Freyer Memorial Lecture. Ir Med J. 1977;70(17):517–22. PubMed PMID: 338549.
27. Keynes EL. The control of haemorrhage after prostatectomy. Ann Surg. 1892;16:454–60.
28. Harris HS. Prostatectomy with complete closure. Med J Aust. 1928;11:288–98.
29. Harris HS. Suprapubic prostatectomy with closure. Br J Urol. 1929;11:285–9.
30. Hryntschak T. Suprapubic transvesical prostatectomy with primary closure of the bladder; improved technic and latest results. J Int Coll Surg. 1951;15(3):366–8. PubMed PMID: 14824592.
31. Millin T. Retropubic prostatectomy; a new extravesical technique; report of 20 cases. Lancet. 1945;2(6380):693–6.
32. White JW. The results of double castration in the hypertrophy of the prostate. Ann Surg. 1895;22:1–3.
33. Murphy LJT. The history of urology. Charles C. Thomas: Springfield; 1972.
34. Abrams P. New words for old: lower urinary tract symptoms for "prostatism". BMJ (Clin Res). 1994;308(6934):929–30. PubMed PMID: 8173393. Pubmed Central PMCID: PMC2539789. Epub 1994/04/09. eng.
35. Abrams P, Feneley RCL, Torrens MJ. Urodynamics. Springer Verlag: Berlin; 1984. p. 6–25.
36. Berry SJ, Coffey DS, Walsh PC, Ewing LL. The development of human benign prostatic hyperplasia with age. J Urol. 1984;132(3):474–9. PubMed PMID: 6206240. Epub 1984/09/01. eng.
37. Denis L, McConnell J, Khoury S, et al. Recommendations of the International Scientific Committee: The evaluation and treatment of lower urinary tract symptoms (LUTS) suggestive of benign prostatic obstruction. In: Denis L, Griffiths K, (eds.). Proceedings of the Fourth

International Consultation on Benign Prostatic Hyperplasia. Health Publications Ltd.: United Kingdom; 1998; 669–84.
38. Roehrborn CG. Focus on lower urinary tract symptoms: nomenclature, diagnosis, and treatment options: highlights from the 5th international consultation on benign prostatic hyperplasia June 25–27, 2000, Paris, France. Rev Urol. 2001;3(3):139–45. PubMed PMID: 16985706. Pubmed Central PMCID: PMC1476056. Epub 2006/09/21. eng.
39. Abrams P, Torrens MJ, Feneley RCL, Cardozo L, Fall M, Griffiths D, et al. The standardisation of terminology of lower urinary tract function: report from the Standardisation Sub-committee of the International Continence Society. Neurourol Urodyn. 2002;21(2):167–78. PubMed PMID: 11857671. Epub 2002/02/22. eng.
40. Abrams P, D'ancona C, Griffiths D, et al. Lower Urinary Tract Symptom: Etiology, Patient Assessment and Predicting Outcome from Therapy. In: Mcconnell J, Abrams P, Denis L, Khoury S, Roehrborn C, (eds.). Male lower urinary tract dysfunction. Evaluation and management. Health Publications: Paris; 2006; 71–142.
41. Chapple CR, Roehrborn CG. A shifted paradigm for the further understanding, evaluation, and treatment of lower urinary tract symptoms in men: focus on the bladder. Eur Urol. 2006;49(4):651–8. PubMed PMID: 16530611. Epub 2006/03/15. eng.
42. Oelke M, Bachmann A, Descazeaud A, Emberton M, Gravas S, Michel MC, et al. Guidelines on the management of male lower urinary tract symptoms (LUTS), incl. benign prostatic obstruction (BPO): European Association of Urology. 2012; 6–8.

Chapter 2
Epidemiology and Pathophysiology of LUTS/BPO

Alberto Briganti and Giorgio Gandaglia

Abstract The prevalence of benign prostatic hyperplasia (BPH) is strongly related to age, ranging from 8 % in men in their 50s to roughly 90 % in men older than 80 years. Although aging represents the strongest risk factor for this, chronic progressive disease, obesity, and metabolic syndrome have been recently shown to be associated with an increased risk of BPH.

The etiology of BPH is still largely unsolved. However, tissue remodeling together with hormonal alterations and chronic inflammation have been recently proposed to be involved in its pathogenesis. The onset of symptoms is determined by prostatic enlargement, which consequently leads to bladder outlet obstruction and changes in the detrusor muscle function, finally resulting in LUTS.

Keywords Benign prostatic hyperplasia • Lower urinary tract symptoms • Epidemiology • Pathophysiology • Risk factors

Epidemiology of BPH and LUTS

Benign prostatic hyperplasia (BPH) is a histological diagnosis defined by the presence of abnormal proliferation of smooth muscle and epithelial cells in prostatic tissues that clinically translates into benign prostatic enlargement (BPE) or obstruction (BPO). Interestingly, BPH is a progressive disease characterized by prostate enlargement, which might subsequently determine the onset of lower urinary symptoms (LUTS).

A. Briganti (✉) • G. Gandaglia
Department of Urology, Urological Research Institute,
Vita-Salute San Raffaele University, Via Olgettina 58,
20132 Milan, Italy
e-mail: briganti.alberto@hsr.it

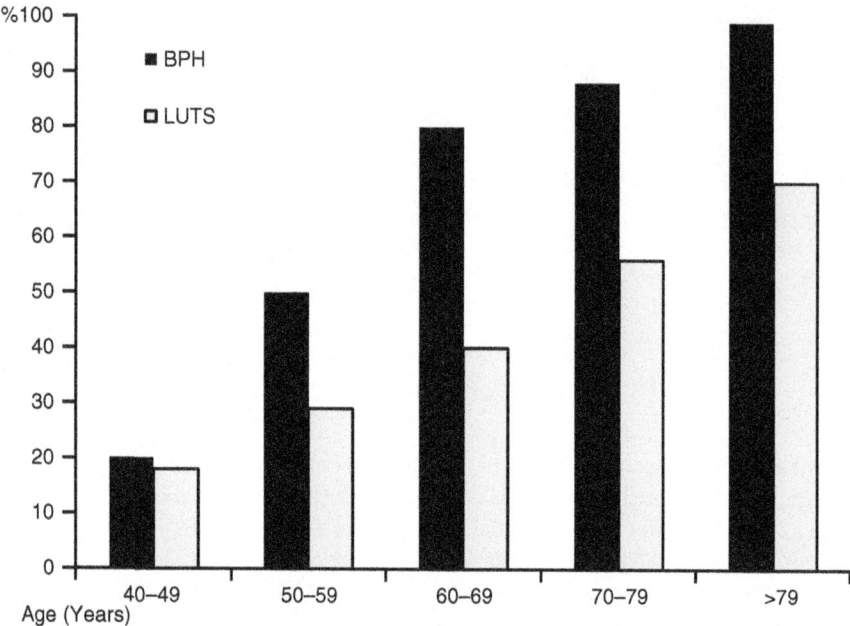

Fig. 2.1 Prevalence of pathological benign prostatic hyperplasia (*BPH*) and lower urinary tract symptoms (*LUTS*) assessed by validated questionnaires stratified by decade of life (Data from Berry et al. [1], Homma et al. [5], Parsons et al. [9])

BPH and LUTS Prevalence

During the past years, several studies assessed the prevalence of BPH, highlighting the role of age in BPH development and LUTS onset. Figure 2.1 depicts the prevalence of these pathological conditions in the general population stratified by age.

The pioneering autopsy study by Berry et al. [1] clearly showed that the incidence of pathological BPH is strongly related to age. Particularly, it has been shown that the normal prostate weights 20 g in individuals aged 21–30 years. No men younger than 30 had BPH. However, the prevalence of BPH increased from 8 to 50 % in individuals in their 40s and 50s, respectively. Men older than 80 years had the highest prevalence of BPH (roughly 90 %) [1, 2].

As previously reported, the clinical manifestation of BPH is commonly represented by LUTS. Several population-based studies evaluated the prevalence of LUTS using validated questionnaires. Particularly, the International Prostatic Symptom Score (IPSS) is a useful tool to stratify patients according to symptom severity [3]. Indeed, patients can be classified in those with no or mild (IPSS ≤7), moderate (IPSS from 8 to 20), and greater-severe symptoms (IPSS ≥21) [4].

Interestingly, also the prevalence of LUTS has been shown to increase with age. In this context, several studies reported that it ranges from 15 % to roughly 60 % in men in their 40s and 70s, respectively [5–8]. Particularly, a large population-based study by Homma et al. evaluated the prevalence of LUTS defined according to the IPSS among 7,588 men in 9 Asian countries and 146 men in Australia. The findings of this study showed that 56 % of men aged 70–79 years had moderate to severe symptoms [5].

These results are in line with what was previously reported by other population-based studies in Europe and North America [6, 8]. In this context, a longitudinal survey of an unselected population of men aged 40–79 years performed in Olmsted, Minnesota (USA), showed that prevalence of moderate to severe symptoms was 13 % in individuals aged 40–49, increasing to 28 % in men older than 70 and rising to approximately 50 % by the eight decade of life [6]. Moreover, LUTS have been shown to affect more than 70 % of men older than 80 years [9].

Interestingly, also the detrimental effects of LUTS on health-related quality of life and on the inability to perform daily activities have been shown to increase with aging and with severity of symptoms [10].

A cross-sectional study of 611 Norwegian men aged 55–70 years showed that prostate volume tended to increase with age [11]. Similarly, a large cross-sectional study performed in Andalusia, Spain, included 1,106 men 40 years or older and estimated the prevalence of BPH according to prostate size measured by TRUS [12]. Interestingly, while mean prostate volume was 23.4 ml in individuals aged 40–49 years, it reached 41.9 ml in men older than 70 years. Accordingly, this study showed that also the transition zone volume increased with age. These findings are in line with what was recently reported in a community-based study including 1,000 men between 40 and 70 years old recruited from the Shanghai community [13]. Again, the authors were able to show a statistical increase in prostate size between each age group. Similar results were obtained when prostate volume was assessed by pelvic magnetic resonance imaging [14].

Finally, a community-based study performed in more than 2,000 individuals 40–79 years old reported that the maximum urinary flow rate decreases from 20 ml/s in men in their 40s to 11.5 ml/s in men in their 70s [15]. Taken together, these findings confirm the increased prevalence of BPH and LUTS with advancing age.

Economic Impact of BPH and LUTS

The high prevalence of BPH determines important health-care system and social costs. Indeed, the economic burden of BPH is related to direct medical costs related to diagnosis and treatment, indirect costs associated with lost work time, and intangible costs associated with reduced quality of life. It has been estimated that the direct costs of medical services to diagnose and treat BPH in the United States were approximately 1.1 billion of USD in 2000 [16]. Moreover, as previously reported, BPH affects up to 50 % of men in their working age. In this population, BPH-related periods of disabilities, diagnosis, and treatment procedures have been estimated to be responsible of up to 38 million hours of lost productivity [16].

From an economic point of view, these data are crucial. Indeed, since the prevalence of BPH and LUTS increases with aging, the economic and social burden of BPH is only likely to increase in the future [17].

Risk Factors for BPH Development

As previously reported, aging represents the most significant risk factor for BPH and LUTS. Race, smoking, alcohol intake, and sexual activity have been hypothesized to increase the risk of BPH. However, evidence is scarce and conflicting regarding their role in prostatic enlargement, and their impact on BPH and LUTS is still poorly understood.

Conversely, the relationship between BPH and obesity, metabolic syndrome, and body mass index (BMI) has been widely assessed. Patients with BMI ≥35 kg/m^2 had higher risk of harboring large prostate volume (>40 ml) and of developing LUTS (IPSS ≥15) compared to those with BMI <25 kg/m^2 [18, 19]. Moreover, men with an obese waist circumference (>109 cm) were at higher risk of being surgically treated for BPH as compared to not obese individuals. In this context, metabolic syndrome, diabetes, and hypertension might predispose patients to BPH and/or LUTS [19, 20]. From a clinical point of view, these data clearly indicate that modification of lifestyle and physical activity may be of benefit to treat or prevent LUTS.

Pathophysiology of BPH and LUTS

Benign prostatic hyperplasia is defined by an abnormal proliferation of epithelial and stromal cells. This proliferation determines an enlargement of the transition zone and the development of nodules in the periurethral region of the prostate [21]. Prostatic enlargement leads to an increase in urethral resistance, resulting in compensatory changes of the detrusor muscle. These alterations in prostate and bladder physiology might consequently lead to the onset of LUTS.

The Etiology of BPH

Several mechanisms have been proposed to be implicated in the pathophysiology of BPH. Although it is well recognized that the increase of prostatic cell number is primarily related to an imbalance in cell proliferation and cell death or apoptosis, the etiology of BPH is still largely unresolved and remains uncertain in some aspects.

Several mechanisms seem to be implicated in the etiology of BPH.

First, a significant tissue-remodeling process in the aging prostate has been hypothesized. Particularly, a decrease of apoptotic activity has been suggested as a key cofactor in BPH pathogenesis and progression in aging males. Indeed, the apoptotic index of the secretory and basal cells of the prostate is lower in BPH compared to normal tissue [22]. This might be related to a certain dysregulation in several growth stimulatory and inhibitory factors involved in the homeostasis of prostatic tissue. For example, tumor growth factor (TGF)-β regulates proliferation, growth arrest, differentiation, and apoptosis of prostatic cells. Since TGF-β is an inhibitor of epithelial cell proliferation in several tissues, a decrease of its expression might reduce the physiological cell death rate, leading to cell proliferation, that might subsequently result in hyperplasia [23].

Second, since prostate is mainly composed by androgen-dependent tissue, a key role of hormonal alterations in the development of BPH has been proposed. In this context, dihydrotestosterone (DHT) is considered the most potent androgen within the prostatic tissue because of its high affinity with androgen receptors. Several evidences support a role of androgens in the pathogenesis of BPH. First, development and growth of prostatic tissue require the presence of testicular androgen during childhood, puberty, and aging [24]. Second, androgen withdrawal might lead to a decrease in protein synthesis and to a subsequent involution of hyperplastic tissues [25]. Third, inhibitors of 5α-reductase, the enzyme which converts testosterone to DHT, are able to lead to a significant reduction of prostate volume and prevent BPH progression [26].

Taken together, these evidences support the hypothesis that the levels of tissue androgens might have a role in the pathogenesis of BPH. Nonetheless, although several studies investigated the relationship between plasma testosterone levels, BPH development, and prostate volume, their results have been inconsistent [23]. Conversely, prospective studies showed that higher serum DHT was associated with an increased risk of BPH [27, 28]. In addition, high testosterone-to-DHT ratios have been shown to decrease the risk of BPH. Thus, it has been hypothesized that patients with higher DHT levels or DHT-to-testosterone ratios might have higher 5α-reductase activity and thus they could be at higher risk of developing BPH [28]. Taken together, all these data seem to suggest that androgens seem to play at least a permissive role in prostate growth.

A role of estrogens in BPH development has also been proposed. Indeed, in aging males, the estrogenic stimulation of the prostatic tissue might lead to the reactivation of epithelial and stromal prostatic cell growth [29, 30]. Interestingly, while androgen levels decrease gradually with aging, estrogen levels remain constant, thus increasing estrogen-to-androgen ratios [31, 32]. In this context, a relationship between estrogens and BPH development has been proposed. Particularly, in older men with high testosterone levels, estradiol has been shown to be significantly associated with increased prostate volume [31]. These findings suggest that estrogen and androgen might play a synergistic effect in BPH development.

Recently, the role of chronic inflammation in the pathogenesis of BPH has emerged. The origin of inflammation still needs to be elucidated. Different sources of prostatic inflammation have been proposed, including bacterial infections, viruses, sexually transmitted organisms, autoimmune response, and urine reflux [33]. The persistence of one or the combination of two or more of these stimuli leads to chronic inflammation. This pathological condition might then contribute to tissue injury, activating cytokine release and increasing the concentration of growth factors, thus creating a local vicious cycle. In this context, the upregulation of pro-inflammatory cytokines has been widely reported in prostatic tissues of patients affected by BPH [34–39]. Particularly, several studies showed an increase in the expression of IL-15, IL-17, interferon-γ, and IL-8 [34–39]. Interestingly, IL-8 has been proposed as a link between chronic prostate inflammation and the development of BPH. This cytokine is produced by epithelial prostate cells and can induce the expression of FGF-2, a potent stromal and epithelial growth factor, and consequently promote the abnormal proliferation of prostatic cells [39]. Local hypoxia may also play a role in the pathophysiology of BPH leading to release of ROS, which can promote neovascularization and growth factor release [40]. These growth factors may interact not only with inflammatory cells but also with the stromal and epithelial cells of the prostate, leading to prostatic enlargement. Taken together, these data support the hypothesis that tissue damage, hypoxia, and chronic process of wound healing lead to a persistent stimulation of stromal and epithelial prostatic tissues, potentially resulting in BPH.

Finally, metabolic syndrome represents a well-established risk factor for the development of BPH. In this context, insulin resistance with secondary hyperinsulinemia has been proposed to have a trophic effect on prostatic tissue and thus to be involved in the development of BPH [41]. High insulin levels might also increase sympathetic nerve activity, increasing prostate smooth muscle tone and thus leading to an increase in urethral resistance. Moreover, insulin can interfere with sex hormone levels, increasing consequently prostate tissue proliferation. Indeed, higher insulin levels might stimulate androgen and estrogen synthesis, which in turn have a stimulatory effect on prostate gland growth. Moreover, diabetes is associated with a reduction in plasma levels of sex hormone-binding globulin, which increases the availability of androgens and estrogens [41]. Metabolic syndrome has also been associated with systemic inflammation and chronic oxidative stress. Interestingly, inflammation might represent a common link between metabolic syndrome and BPH pathogenesis. Indeed, cytokine release and oxidative stress related to metabolic syndrome might contribute to the chronic inflammatory pattern in BPH patients, resulting in wound healing and consequent proliferation of prostatic tissues [42–44] (Fig. 2.2).

BPH and LUTS Pathogenesis

Benign prostatic hyperplasia is a pathological condition characterized by an increase in the number of prostatic cells, and not in their size. Thus, it should be considered a hyperplastic process. Benign prostatic hyperplasia initially leads to the development of periurethral and transitional zone nodules. Particularly, while transition zone nodules represent the proliferation of glandular tissue, periurethral nodules are mainly composed by stromal cells [45]. Interestingly, although in the earlier phase of the disease BPH is characterized by an increase in the number of nodules, in the

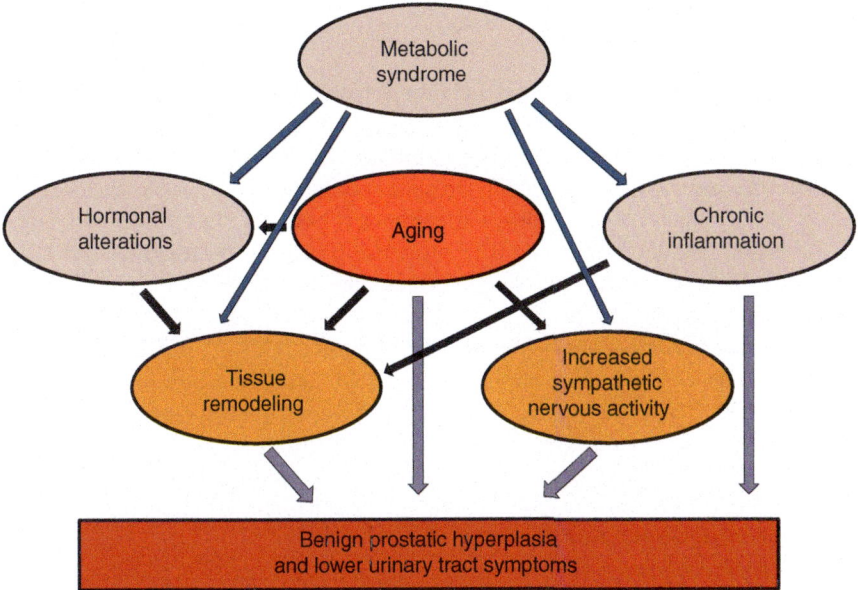

Fig. 2.2 Relationship between age, metabolic syndrome, hormonal alterations, chronic prostatic inflammation, tissue remodeling, and sympathetic nervous activity in the pathogenesis of benign prostatic hyperplasia (BPH) and lower urinary tract symptoms (LUTS)

later phase, a significant increase in nodule volume occurs [23]. This leads to prostatic enlargement and thus increases urethral resistance, consequently resulting in compensatory alterations of detrusor muscle and in the onset of LUTS.

The process of not only nodule development and glandular enlargement but also prostatic smooth muscle tone has a role in the pathogenesis of LUTS. Indeed, prostatic smooth muscle is controlled by the adrenergic nervous system, and its stimulation results in a significant increase of urethral resistance. This has also been confirmed by the use of α-receptor blockers in the management of BPH. Taken together, these evidences raised the hypothesis that autonomic nervous system overactivity might be involved in LUTS onset in patients with BPH [46, 47].

We can therefore conclude that bladder outlet obstruction has three different components. The first consists of prostatic enlargement related to BPH, which leads to a static urethral obstruction. The second includes the dynamic component of obstruction related to increased prostatic muscular tone determined by autonomic nervous activity (namely, the sympathetic tone). These changes in micturition physiology lead to bladder adaptive response. Particularly, the initial response of the detrusor to bladder outlet increased resistance is hypertrophy. However, the increase in smooth muscle mass is associated with changes in muscle cell phenotypes, which finally lead to abnormal collagen production and detrusor instability [48]. The third is represented by the inflammatory component which may act as a link between the static and the dynamic parts.

Natural History of BPH/LUTS

As previously reported, BPH and LUTS are increasingly prevalent conditions in aging males. Although the rate of enlargement varies at individual level, prostate growth rate peaks at 4.15 cc/year for individuals aged 56–65 years and then rapidly declines for older men [49]. Not only prostate volume but also LUTS prevalence has been shown to increase with aging. Furthermore, it has been reported that older men are at higher risk of experiencing BPH progression (namely, deterioration of LUTS, decreased peak flow rate, increased prostate volume, acute urinary retention, and BPH-related surgery).

The Olmsted County study well describes the natural history of BPH in a cohort of 2,115 men aged 40–79 years [6, 50]. This longitudinal study of community-dwelling men clearly showed an increase in LUTS severity with aging. Particularly, the prevalence of moderate to severe LUTS ranged from 26 to 46 % in men aged 40–49 and 70–79 years, respectively [6]. The mean increase in the IPSS has been estimated in 0.18 points per year. Accordingly, a consistent decline in peak urinary flow rate was also observed [50].

When the occurrence of acute urinary retention was examined, this longitudinal study showed an increase in the incidence of this pathological condition from 1 % in individuals aged 40–40 years to 9 % among those 70–79 years old [51]. Interestingly, older age and the severity of LUTS were significantly associated with higher risk of acute urinary retention. These findings were also confirmed by the evaluation of men included in the placebo group of prospective randomized clinical trials. Although the results of these studies are limited by the stringent inclusion criteria and biased by the administration of the placebo itself, they clearly show symptom deterioration and increasing incidence of acute urinary retention with aging [52, 53].

Finally, also the need for surgical treatment for BPH has been shown to be strongly age related. Particularly, in the Olmsted County study, the rates of BPH-related surgery ranged from 0.1 to 9.5 % in individuals aged 40–49 years and in those 70–79 years old, respectively [54]. Similarly, among men enrolled in the placebo arm of the Medical Therapy of Prostatic Symptoms (MTOPS) study, the need for BPH-related surgery increased with aging [52]. Taken together, these evidences clearly demonstrate that BPH is a progressive disease.

References

1. Berry SJ, Coffey DS, Walsh PC, Ewing LL. The development of human benign prostatic hyperplasia with age. J Urol. 1984;132(3):474–9.
2. Boyle P. New insights into the epidemiology and natural history of benign prostatic hyperplasia. Prog Clin Biol Res. 1994;386:3–18.
3. Barry MJ, Fowler Jr FJ, O'Leary MP, et al. The American Urological Association symptom index for benign prostatic hyperplasia. The Measurement Committee of the American Urological Association. J Urol. 1992;148(5):1549–57; discussion 64.
4. Homma Y, Kawabe K, Tsukamoto T, et al. Estimate criteria for diagnosis and severity in benign prostatic hyperplasia. Int J Urol. 1996;3(4):261–6.

5. Homma Y, Kawabe K, Tsukamoto T, et al. Epidemiologic survey of lower urinary tract symptoms in Asia and Australia using the international prostate symptom score. Int J Urol. 1997;4(1):40–6.
6. Chute CG, Panser LA, Girman CJ, et al. The prevalence of prostatism: a population-based survey of urinary symptoms. J Urol. 1993;150(1):85–9.
7. Roehrborn CG. The epidemiology of acute urinary retention in benign prostatic hyperplasia. Rev Urol. 2001 Fall;3(4):187–92.
8. Bosch JL, Kranse R, van Mastrigt R, Schroder FH. Reasons for the weak correlation between prostate volume and urethral resistance parameters in patients with prostatism. J Urol. 1995;153(3 Pt 1):689–93.
9. Parsons JK, Bergstrom J, Silberstein J, Barrett-Connor E. Prevalence and characteristics of lower urinary tract symptoms in men aged > or = 80 years. Urology. 2008;72(2):318–21.
10. Girman CJ, Jacobsen SJ, Tsukamoto T, et al. Health-related quality of life associated with lower urinary tract symptoms in four countries. Urology. 1998;51(3):428–36.
11. Overland GB, Vatten L, Rhodes T, et al. Lower urinary tract symptoms, prostate volume and uroflow in Norwegian community men. Eur Urol. 2001;39(1):36–41.
12. Chicharro-Molero JA, Burgos-Rodriguez R, Sanchez-Cruz JJ, del Rosal-Samaniego JM, Rodero-Carcia P, Rodriguez-Vallejo JM. Prevalence of benign prostatic hyperplasia in Spanish men 40 years old or older. J Urol. 1998;159(3):878–82.
13. Zhang SJ, Qian HN, Zhao Y, et al. Relationship between age and prostate size. Asian J Androl. 2013;15(1):116–20.
14. Roehrborn CG, McConnell J, Bonilla J, et al. Serum prostate specific antigen is a strong predictor of future prostate growth in men with benign prostatic hyperplasia. PROSCAR long-term efficacy and safety study. J Urol. 2000;163(1):13–20.
15. Girman CJ, Panser LA, Chute CG, et al. Natural history of prostatism: urinary flow rates in a community-based study. J Urol. 1993;150(3):887–92.
16. Wei JT, Calhoun E, Jacobsen SJ. Urologic diseases in America project: benign prostatic hyperplasia. J Urol. 2005;173(4):1256–61.
17. Kirby RS, Kirby M, Fitzpatrick JM. Benign prostatic hyperplasia: counting the cost of its management. BJU Int. 2010;105(7):901–2.
18. Issa MM, Regan TS. Medical therapy for benign prostatic hyperplasia – present and future impact. Am J Manag Care. 2007;13 Suppl 1:S4–9.
19. Abdollah F, Briganti A, Suardi N, et al. Metabolic syndrome and benign prostatic hyperplasia: evidence of a potential relationship, hypothesized etiology, and prevention. Korean J Urol. 2011;52(8):507–16.
20. De Nunzio C, Aronson W, Freedland SJ, Giovannucci E, Parsons JK. The correlation between metabolic syndrome and prostatic diseases. Eur Urol. 2012;61(3):560–70.
21. McNeal J. Pathology of benign prostatic hyperplasia. Insight into etiology. Urol Clin North Am. 1990;17(3):477–86.
22. Zhao Y, Peng J, Zheng L, Yu W, Jin J. Transforming growth factor beta1 mediates apoptotic activity of angiotensin II type I receptor blocker on prostate epithelium in vitro. Prostate. 2010;70(8):899–905.
23. Roehrborn CG. Pathology of benign prostatic hyperplasia. Int J Impot Res. 2008;20 Suppl 3:S11–8.
24. Wilson JD, Roehrborn C. Long-term consequences of castration in men: lessons from the Skoptzy and the eunuchs of the Chinese and Ottoman courts. J Clin Endocrinol Metab. 1999;84(12):4324–31.
25. Stone NN, Clejan SJ. Response of prostate volume, prostate-specific antigen, and testosterone to flutamide in men with benign prostatic hyperplasia. J Androl. 1991;12(6):376–80.
26. Jeong YB, Kwon KS, Kim SD, Kim HJ. Effect of discontinuation of 5alpha-reductase inhibitors on prostate volume and symptoms in men with BPH: a prospective study. Urology. 2009;73(4):802–6.
27. Parsons JK, Palazzi-Churas K, Bergstrom J, Barrett-Connor E. Prospective study of serum dihydrotestosterone and subsequent risk of benign prostatic hyperplasia in community dwelling men: the Rancho Bernardo Study. J Urol. 2010;184(3):1040–4.

28. Liao CH, Li HY, Chung SD, Chiang HS, Yu HJ. Significant association between serum dihydrotestosterone level and prostate volume among Taiwanese men aged 40–79 years. Aging Male. 2012;15(1):28–33.
29. Thomas JA, Keenan EJ. Effects of estrogens on the prostate. J Androl. 1994;15(2):97–9.
30. Prins GS, Huang L, Birch L, Pu Y. The role of estrogens in normal and abnormal development of the prostate gland. Ann N Y Acad Sci. 2006;1089:1–13.
31. Roberts RO, Jacobson DJ, Rhodes T, Klee GG, Leiber MM, Jacobsen SJ. Serum sex hormones and measures of benign prostatic hyperplasia. Prostate. 2004;61(2):124–31.
32. Vermeulen A, Kaufman JM, Goemaere S, van Pottelberg I. Estradiol in elderly men. Aging Male. 2002;5(2):98–102.
33. De Marzo AM, Platz EA, Sutcliffe S, et al. Inflammation in prostate carcinogenesis. Nat Rev Cancer. 2007;7(4):256–69.
34. De Nunzio C, Kramer G, Marberger M, et al. The controversial relationship between benign prostatic hyperplasia and prostate cancer: the role of inflammation. Eur Urol. 2011;60(1):106–17.
35. Steiner GE, Newman ME, Paikl D, et al. Expression and function of pro-inflammatory interleukin IL-17 and IL-17 receptor in normal, benign hyperplastic, and malignant prostate. Prostate. 2003;56(3):171–82.
36. Steiner GE, Stix U, Handisurya A, et al. Cytokine expression pattern in benign prostatic hyperplasia infiltrating T cells and impact of lymphocytic infiltration on cytokine mRNA profile in prostatic tissue. Lab Invest. 2003;83(8):1131–46.
37. Handisurya A, Steiner GE, Stix U, et al. Differential expression of interleukin-15, a proinflammatory cytokine and T-cell growth factor, and its receptor in human prostate. Prostate. 2001;49(4):251–62.
38. Royuela M, de Miguel MP, Ruiz A, et al. Interferon-gamma and its functional receptors overexpression in benign prostatic hyperplasia and prostatic carcinoma: parallelism with c-myc and p53 expression. Eur Cytokine Netw. 2000;11(1):119–27.
39. Giri D, Ittmann M. Interleukin-8 is a paracrine inducer of fibroblast growth factor 2, a stromal and epithelial growth factor in benign prostatic hyperplasia. Am J Pathol. 2001;159(1):139–47.
40. Wang L, Yang JR, Yang LY, Liu ZT. Chronic inflammation in benign prostatic hyperplasia: implications for therapy. Med Hypotheses. 2008;70(5):1021–3.
41. Sarma AV, Parsons JK, McVary K, Wei JT. Diabetes and benign prostatic hyperplasia/lower urinary tract symptoms – what do we know? J Urol. 2009;182(6 Suppl):S32–7.
42. Alexandraki K, Piperi C, Kalofoutis C, Singh J, Alaveras A, Kalofoutis A. Inflammatory process in type 2 diabetes: the role of cytokines. Ann N Y Acad Sci. 2006;1084:89–117.
43. Gustafson B, Hammarstedt A, Andersson CX, Smith U. Inflamed adipose tissue: a culprit underlying the metabolic syndrome and atherosclerosis. Arterioscler Thromb Vasc Biol. 2007;27(11):2276–83.
44. Murdolo G, Smith U. The dysregulated adipose tissue: a connecting link between insulin resistance, type 2 diabetes mellitus and atherosclerosis. Nutr Metab Cardiovasc Dis. 2006;16 Suppl 1:S35–8.
45. McNeal JE. Origin and evolution of benign prostatic enlargement. Invest Urol. 1978;15(4):340–5.
46. Gacci M, Eardley I, Giuliano F, et al. Critical analysis of the relationship between sexual dysfunctions and lower urinary tract symptoms due to benign prostatic hyperplasia. Eur Urol. 2011;60(4):809–25.
47. McVary KT, Rademaker A, Lloyd GL, Gann P. Autonomic nervous system overactivity in men with lower urinary tract symptoms secondary to benign prostatic hyperplasia. J Urol. 2005;174(4 Pt 1):1327–433.
48. Anumanthan G, Tanaka ST, Adams CM, et al. Bladder stromal loss of transforming growth factor receptor II decreases fibrosis after bladder obstruction. J Urol. 2009;182(4 Suppl):1775–80.

49. Williams AM, Simon I, Landis PK, et al. Prostatic growth rate determined from MRI data: age-related longitudinal changes. J Androl. 1999;20(4):474–80.
50. Roberts RO, Jacobsen SJ, Jacobson DJ, Rhodes T, Girman CJ, Lieber MM. Longitudinal changes in peak urinary flow rates in a community based cohort. J Urol. 2000;163(1):107–13.
51. Jacobsen SJ, Jacobson DJ, Girman CJ, et al. Natural history of prostatism: risk factors for acute urinary retention. J Urol. 1997;158(2):481–7.
52. McConnell JD, Roehrborn CG, Bautista OM, et al. The long-term effect of doxazosin, finasteride, and combination therapy on the clinical progression of benign prostatic hyperplasia. N Engl J Med. 2003;349(25):2387–98.
53. Roehrborn CG. Alfuzosin 10 mg once daily prevents overall clinical progression of benign prostatic hyperplasia but not acute urinary retention: results of a 2-year placebo-controlled study. BJU Int. 2006;97(4):734–41.
54. Jacobsen SJ, Jacobson DJ, Girman CJ, et al. Treatment for benign prostatic hyperplasia among community dwelling men: the Olmsted County study of urinary symptoms and health status. J Urol. 1999;162(4):1301–6.

Chapter 3
Assessing LUTS/BPO: What Is the Evidence?

Cosimo De Nunzio and Riccardo Autorino

Abstract Lower urinary tract symptoms (LUTS) can be caused by multiple conditions that include benign prostatic obstruction (BPO) as the most important and frequent cause in male patients. During the past decade, the pathophysiology of LUTS/BPO has been completely revisited and many changes in the diagnosis and medical and surgical management of LUTS have evolved and are available in clinical practice. Several national and international urological associations have developed clinical guidelines and algorithms to help diagnosing and managing patients with LUTS/BPO. Patient assessment aims at establishing the pathophysiology of LUTS in the individual subject and includes recommended tests (medical history, quantification of symptoms and bother, physical examination, urinalysis, biochemical tests, frequency volume chart) to be performed in all patients with LUTS/BPO and optional tests (uroflowmetry, post-void residual volume (PVR), urinary tract imaging, pressure–flow studies, and endoscopy of the lower urinary tract) to be considered for the specialized management. The implementation and validation of the available algorithms and guidelines could improve patients' management and patients/physician communication and finally reduce the number of unneeded examinations in patients with LUTS/BPO reducing the social costs of the disease.

C. De Nunzio (✉)
Department of Urology, Ospedale Sant'Andrea,
University "La Sapienza", Rome, Italy

YAU-EAU BPH Group, Italy
e-mail: cosimodenunzio@virgilio.it

R. Autorino
Urology Unit, Second University of Naples, Naples, Italy

YAU-EAU BPH Group, Italy
e-mail: ricautor@gmail.com

The aim of this chapter is to summarize the current evidence on the diagnostic work-up for the management of patients with LUTS/BPO and to highlight differences between different international guidelines or algorithms.

Keywords Prostate • Prostatic hyperplasia • BPH • LUTS • Diagnosis • Disease management

Introduction

Lower urinary tract symptoms (LUTS) in adult male have been traditionally attributed to the enlargement of the prostate gland. However, during the last decade, the causal link between the prostate and the pathogenesis of LUTS has come into question. Although benign prostatic enlargement (BPE) can significantly contribute to the onset of LUTS in a proportion of men over 40 years of age, other metabolic, neurological, inflammatory, and anatomical factors should be considered [4] and (EAU guidelines 2012).

Considering that patients seek medical advice for LUTS rather than the underlying anatomical condition, an accurate assessment of patients with LUTS should take into account the possible relationship between BPE, BPO, and LUTS but also to all the other potential causing factors.

During the past two decades, the 6th International Consultation on New Developments in Prostate Cancer and Prostatic Diseases, the European Association of Urology (EAU), the American Urological Association (AUA), and the National Institute for Clinical Excellence (NICE) in the United Kingdom have developed and updated clinical practice guidelines (CPGs) and algorithms, with the purpose to implement a cost-effective management of LUTS/BPO [10, 18–20]. Notwithstanding all guidelines stem from a common knowledge base, their recommendations may differ because of variation in experts' opinion, national health system resources, reimbursement issues, etc. [30]. Primary evaluation of patients can be performed by general practitioners and office- or hospital-based urologist; in general, academic and urban urologists tend to be more compliant with the CPGs, making the management of LUTS/BPO more uniform [10]. In daily clinical practice, the management of LUTS is still related to physician and patient shared decision-making and to local policies of individual countries (Table 3.1).

History and Physical Examination

History and physical examination aim at diagnosing concomitant conditions of the bladder, the central nervous system, or other organs that may be responsible for LUTS beyond benign and malignant disorders of the prostate [30]. All available guidelines highly recommend that a detailed medical history should always

Table 3.1 A summary of the recommendations for diagnostic testing in the basic management of men with BPH/LUTS

	6th International Consultation on Prostatic Diseases 2006 and AUA guidelines 2011	EAU guidelines 2012	NICE recommendations 2009
History and physical examination	R	R	R
Use of symptom score	R	R	R
Urine analysis	R	R	R
Serum creatinine	O	R	O
Serum PSA	O	R	O
Use of a voiding diary	R	R	R
Uroflowmetry	O	R	O
PVR measurement	O	O	O
Imaging urinary tract	NR	R	O
Pressure–flow study	NR	NR	NR
Endoscopy	NR	NR	NR

R recommended, *O* optional, *NR* not recommended

represent the first step in the clinical assessment of patients presenting with LUTS. Medical history should be taken by focusing on the urinary tract and to identify conditions, other than prostate disorders, which may be responsible causes of voiding and storage dysfunction or comorbidities necessitating of more accurate diagnostic tools. An appropriate medical history should focus on the nature and duration of reported genitourinary symptoms, allocating symptoms to the appropriate stage of the bladder cycle, evaluating previous medical and surgical procedures, medications taken by the patient, as well as coexisting diseases, cognitive function, environmental and lifestyle issues (including exercise, smoking, and the type of food/fluid intake), and patients' goals and expectation of treatment [1, 19].

Physical examination is of importance as it allows ruling out conditions that may require immediate treatment and occult disorders that may be responsible for LUTS. A general physical examination with a specific attention to the presence or absence of a distended bladder, excoriation of the genitals (secondary to urinary incontinence), evidence of urethral discharge, anatomical abnormalities (penile curvature, site of urethral meatus, presence and size of both testis), and a focused neurological examination is also highly recommended [1].

Digital rectal examination of the prostate has a low sensitivity and specificity for prostate cancer detection, and it now plays a minor role compared to the pre-PSA and pre-ultrasound era. However, it remains a valid test to diagnose BPE, although it underestimates prostate volume as compared with transrectal ultrasound or magnetic resonance, to rule out acute prostatic inflammation, locally advanced prostate cancer, neurological conditions that may affect anal sphincter tone, and cancer of the lower part of the rectum [1, 5, 25, 29]. Clinical examination also allows ruling out the possible presence of metabolic syndrome, whose association with prostatic disorders has been recently pointed out [8, 13]. Physician should evaluate blood pressure, height, weight, and waist circumference to identify the occurrence of arterial hypertension and define the presence of obesity and particularly of an abdominal obesity.

Questionnaires

Validated questionnaires have been developed to standardize the assessment of patients' symptoms but also to predict the response to treatment and to assess treatment outcome.

Different symptom scores are currently available and have been validated in several languages (IPSS, ICIQMLUTS, DAN-PSS, OAB-q). All of them contain one or more questions about quality of life and symptom bother [29].

The International Prostatic Symptom Score (IPSS)

The American Urological Association score described by Barry and his colleagues has been adopted by the World Health Organization-patronized Consultation on BPH in 1991 as International Prostate Symptom Score (IPSS) and has become the international standard [3, 30]. The IPSS is an 8-question tool (7 symptom questions + 1 quality of life question) designed to be completed by the patients and used to provide the physicians a uniform and reproducible method of assessing symptoms and facilitating comparisons of the results from clinical trials. Each question can be answered on a scale of 0–5 and therefore the total score ranges from 0 to 35. A score from 0 to 8 defines the presence of mild symptoms, 8–19 of moderate symptoms, and 20–35 of severe symptoms [1, 19]. Sub-scores of the voiding and storage symptoms can be also obtained. The IPSS can also be used over time to compare the progression of symptoms and their severity over months and years or to evaluate symptoms response after treatment. A change of at least 3 points is considered the threshold of a clinically relevant change that can be perceived by the patient. Although the IPSS has many advantages as it is self-administered, sensitive to changes, and generalizable to different populations and socioeconomic groups, it presents several limitations. This tool is not disease or condition specific, it does not represent a diagnostic tool for the diagnosis of BPO, and it poorly correlates with other variables such as prostate volume, urinary flow rate, and post-void residual urine. Furthermore, the IPSS does not address urinary incontinence and it may therefore be suboptimal whenever continence is impaired [1, 30]. Notwithstanding all these limitations, the IPSS is the most popular symptom score and it is recommended by almost all the available guidelines for the initial evaluation of patients presenting with LUTS/BPO.

The International Consultation on Incontinence Questionnaire: ICIQ-Male LUTS

The International Consultation on Incontinence Modular Questionnaire was developed following the advice of the International Consultation on Incontinence held in 1998 under the auspices of the World Health Organization and organized by the International Continence Society (ICS) and the International Consultation on Urological Diseases (ICUD). The ICIQ-Male LUTS aimed to overcome some limitations of the IPSS. It was developed from patients with urodynamically investigated BOO. The ICIQ-Male LUTS includes 14 questions: 5 assessing voiding symptoms, 6 assessing incontinence symptoms, and 1 question each on frequency, nocturia, and quality of life; in most of the questions, a scale for the degree of bother is included. This is considered a primary questionnaire for the assessment of the occurrence and bothersomeness of a wide range of LUTS in men including symptoms of incontinence [1].

The ICIQ-Male LUTS is considered as a more conventional tool to evaluate the impact of LUTS on quality of life as it is significantly impacted and impaired by BPH. It has been translated and validated into 30 languages, although it has not yet had the same popularity in clinical practice as has the IPSS [1].

The Danish Prostate Symptom Score (DAN-PSS)

The Danish Prostate Symptom Score (DAN-PSS) was designed in Denmark to diagnose the presence and severity of LUTS and to measure the degree to which men are bothered by each urinary symptom [1]. It was designed for BPH patients with no serious complications and it consists of 12 questions. Each question is graded from 0 to 3, and for each symptom, the bothersomeness is graded from 0 (no problem) to 3 (severe problem). A composite score is defined by the multiplication of the symptom score by the bother score with a total range of 0–108. Thus, severe symptoms with no bother will contribute zero to the total score. The DAN-PSS has been shown to identify patients with LUTS suggestive of BPO and to appropriately identify symptom changes after medical or surgical treatment in patients with LUTS/BPO, although it could not sufficiently predict the success or failure of transurethral prostate resection [1]

The Overactive Bladder Questionnaire (OAB-Q)

The overactive bladder symptom and health-related quality of life questionnaire (OAB-q) is designed to specifically assess the symptom bother and the related quality of life impact of an overactive bladder in both men and women. The questionnaire was developed during the National Overactive Bladder Evaluation

(NOBLE) program in the United States and it contains 33 items (8 on bladder symptoms including urge incontinence and accidental loss of urine and 25 related to the impact of the symptoms on coping, concern/worry, sleep, and social interaction). The OAB-q has been extensively validated in different languages and it has demonstrated reliability, validity, responsiveness in discriminating between continent and incontinent OAB patients, and controls without OAB [6, 7, 27]. The OAB-q has also shown to distinguish patients with varying levels of urge intensity, micturition frequency, and episodes of nocturia. Improvements in OAB-q scales were associated with changes in patient and physician perceptions of treatment benefit. The 19-item short form consists in a six-item symptom bother scale and 13-item health-related quality of life has been also recently developed and validated [6, 7, 27]. Although the OAB-q has not been routinely used or recommended in patients with LUTS/BPO, given the high prevalence of OAB in patients with LUTS/BPO and its substantial negative impact on patients' quality of life, reliable and well-validated measures should be implemented to assess treatment outcomes on these patients.

Urinalysis and Biochemical Testing

Urinalysis

Urinalysis is an inexpensive test, not requiring sophisticated technologies, without side effects, and it is generally recommended by LUTS/BPO guidelines in primary care management. Urinalysis is routinely performed in any setting using dipsticks to identify hematuria, glycosuria, proteinuria, pyuria, specific gravity, and the presence of urinary nitrites and leukocyte esterase. However, a dipstick test, while suggestive of urinary tract infection, is useful as a screening test and abnormal findings need to be confirmed by a midstream specimen of urine (MSU) [19]. Complete urinalysis includes physical, chemical, and microscopic examinations, and although associated with false-positive and false-negative results, it is considered a simple, noninvasive, and cost-effective test to identify patients with urinary tract infection for the presence of leukocyte esterases and nitrites or patients with microscopic hematuria [1]. Since LUTS can be associated to urinary tract infection, bladder carcinoma, and distal urethral or bladder stones, a normal microscopic examination of the urine sediment should make these diagnoses less likely [23].

Blood Tests

Although there is no association between BPE and chronic kidney disease and recent data from the Medical Treatment of Prostate Symptoms (MTOPS) study suggest that the risk of developing de novo renal failure in men with LUTS is less than 1 %, the EAU and most of the available national guidelines still recommend to measure serum creatinine in primary care management [1, 15, 20]. According to these guidelines, the risk of missing a diagnosis of renal failure in patients evaluated for LUTS/BPO could balance the expenditure of screening for renal failure using serum creatinine evaluation [1]. Considering that diabetes and arterial hypertension are the most important cause of elevated serum creatinine in men with proven BPO and renal failure and that they are both key features of the metabolic syndrome recently associated with LUTS and BPH, some authors have suggested to include a metabolic serum screening (glycemia, triglyceridemia, HDL) in the primary care and specialized management of patients with LUTS [1, 8, 12]. On the other side, the NICE recommends to offer men with LUTS a serum creatinine test only if there are any indications of renal impairment (e.g., palpable bladder, nocturnal enuresis, recurrent urinary tract infection, or history of renal stones) [19].

Prostate-specific antigen (PSA) is produced by benign prostatic epithelia cells; although it has been primarily used in the management of prostatic cancer since its introduction in the 1980s, we know that many patients with benign prostatic diseases and LUTS have a raised PSA. An evaluation of PSA in the adult male population is no longer limited to the diagnosis of prostatic cancer, but it could have a role in the management of patients with LUTS/BPO. Serum PSA proved to be a surrogate of prostate volume and has been shown to be a strong predictor of the risk of acute urinary retention and need for surgery in men with BPE. Thus, it can be used to identify patients at risk of BPE progression which could necessitate a specific therapeutic regimen (Combat and MTOPS), Roehrborn et al. [24, 25]. In patients with LUTS, those with a PSA more than 4 ng/ml are significantly associated to have some degree of BPO; conversely, patients with a PSA less than 2 ng/ml have a 33 % chance to be obstructed [1]. Notwithstanding the PSA assessment in male patients with LUTS/BPO is twofold, to screen prostate cancer and to measure a proxy of prostate volume, BPH progression, and response to treatment; its routine use remains controversial. The EAU suggests measuring PSA in men with LUTS and a life expectancy of over 10 years in whom the diagnosis of prostate cancer would change the management of patient's voiding symptoms [22, 30]. The AUA panel recommends that the benefit and risks of PSA testing should be discussed with the patient including its low accuracy for prostate cancer detection and the possible complications associated with prostate biopsy and with the overtreatment of clinically insignificant prostate cancer [2, 10]. According to the NICE group, PSA can be considered optional in primary care management and physician should offer men with LUTS information, advice, and time to decide if they wish to have PSA testing, particularly when LUTS are suggestive of bladder outlet obstruction secondary to BPE or in case of abnormal DRE or when there are concerns about prostate cancer [19].

Frequency–Volume Charts

Frequency–volume charts have become an important part of the evaluation of patients with LUTS/BPO particularly of those who have storage symptoms, such as urinary frequency, incontinence, or nocturia. They are fundamental to analyze day- and nighttime frequency, mean voided volume, total urine output, nocturnal urine output, urgency, and urgency incontinence episodes [19, 29].

The frequency–volume chart (FVC) records the time and volume of each micturition, but a number of different diaries have been defined by the International Continence Society (ICS): The micturition time chart records only the times that voids occur without volumetric data whereas the bladder diary records the time and volume of each micturition and it may also include other data such as incontinence episodes, pad usage, fluid intake, and urgency [19]. The ICS has recommended voiding diaries to be performed for at least 24 h, although, in clinical practice, a period of 3–7 days is usually chosen; most patients find the use of diaries to be acceptable for short periods [19]. Although no clinical or economic studies have evaluated the cost-effectiveness of FVCs in male patients with LUTS/BPO, the NICE recommends the use of FVCs in men with LUTS at the time of their initial and specialized assessment. The EAU guidelines suggest an initial evaluation with FVCs in patients with nocturia or polyuria. FVCs are critical for the evaluation of nocturia as they allow distinguishing between nocturnal overactive bladder and nocturnal polyuria, two common causes of nocturia [1]. Paper diaries have been traditionally used in clinical practice, although recent experiences suggested that the electronic diary is an appropriate alternative to a paper-based method to evaluate patients with LUTS [1]. One possible limitation to the clinical use of FVCs may be related to patients' learning difficulties, dyslexia, blindness, and language barriers or cognitive impairment. In these specific situations, it is advisable to assist the patient during the FVC compilation.

Post-void Residual Urine

The 6th International Consultation on New Developments in Prostate Cancer and Prostatic Diseases considered the determination of post-void residual urine a useful but optional test in the initial diagnostic assessment of patients with LUTS/BPO, although it is considered a recommended test in the specialized management [1].

PVR evaluation aims to diagnose significant residual urine or chronic retention as a possible cause of LUTS or as risk factors of urinary tract infection and acute urinary retention. However, the relation between elevated PVR and UTI is controversial and it is in fact evident only in the pediatric, neurological, diabetic, or elderly patients. There is also no evidence that UTI, renal failure, acute urinary retention, and BPH progression are more common in men with large, chronic residuals [1]. Because of large patient variability, it is not possible to establish a PVR cutoff point for decision-making. The value of 50–100 ml has been considered as a possible lower threshold to define abnormal residual urine and value >300 ml is used to identify patients at risk of unfavorable outcome after LUTS/BPO treatment. PVR can be measured by in and out catheterization, by ultrasonography by measurement of bladder height, width, and length [9], or by using recently portable ultrasound devices for the automated measurement of the volume of urine in the bladder with a concomitant assessment of the bladder mass and detrusor wall thickness, which were introduced (BVM6500 and BVM 9500; Verathon, Bothell, Washington, USA) in the market [31].

Uroflowmetry

Uroflowmetry is a noninvasive test that gives useful information regarding voiding function by measuring the rate of flow of voided urine. It is performed using a flowmeter, a device that measures the quantity of fluid (volume or mass) voided per unit of time; in this case, the measurement is expressed in milliliters per second (ml/s). Patients are instructed to void normally, either sitting or standing, with a comfortably full bladder, and should be provided with private and comfortable surroundings [19]. It can identify patients with abnormal voiding pattern and monitor changes in voiding dynamics over time in watchful waiting programs and follow-up of medical therapy, physical treatment, or surgical therapies. Although the uroflow study is the most commonly performed noninvasive urodynamic test, it does not discriminate BPO from poor detrusor contractility. The sensitivity and specificity of maximum free flow rate (Q_{max}) versus diagnosis of BPO are, respectively, 47 and 70 % for Q_{max} less than 10 ml/s and 82 and 38 % for Q_{max} less than 15 ml/s [1]. The range of likelihood ratios for a positive test for obstruction (LR+) is between 1.6 and 3.8 suggesting that urinary flow rate misdiagnoses a variable proportion of patients as unobstructed when they are obstructed when compared to the suggested standard of LR+=10 for a test with good discriminatory power. The range of likelihood ratios for a negative test for obstruction (LR−) is between 0.03 and 0.5 suggesting that urinary flow rate misdiagnoses a variable proportion of patients as obstructed when they have no obstruction compared to the suggested standard of 0.1 for a test with good discriminatory power [19]. Uroflow studies presented also other limits as variability over repeated test related to patient's learning effect, circadian effect, uroflowmeter artifacts, and intra-observer, interobserver variation from manual correction of uroflow traces. There is also evidence that a single flow rate or a flow rate based upon a voided volume <150 ml is insufficient for reliable interpretation, and several single flow analysis with an adequate voiding volume should be performed to obtain a definitive conclusion [19, 30].

Although the EAU guidelines recommend uroflowmetry in the initial work-up of patients with LUTS/BPO, its role is still controversial and debated. In particular, the NICE and the 6th International Consultation on New Developments in Prostate Cancer and Prostatic Diseases recommend uroflowmetry evaluation only in the specialized management of patients with LUTS/BPO [1, 19, 20].

Imaging

Urinary Tract Ultrasound

Imaging of upper and lower urinary tract system has been used for several years as part of the diagnostic assessment of men with LUTS/BPO. Although renal ultrasound is a noninvasive, widely used test in the assessment of many urological problems, involves no radiation, and is highly acceptable to patients, nowadays, its routine use has not been considered as a first-line test in almost LUTS/BPO diagnosis guidelines. Many urologists do not take images of the upper urinary tract routinely because tumors and kidney stones or failure are not more frequent in men with LUTS related to BPH than in healthy men [30]. However, according to the NICE recommendations, renal ultrasound should be considered as the imaging modality of the upper urinary tract in patients with LUTS/BPH and a history of chronic retention, hematuria, recurrent urinary tract infection, sterile pyuria, profound symptoms, or pain [19].

Imaging of the lower urinary tract includes bladder and prostate. Bladder imaging is usually performed for evaluating PVR but also provides information regarding possible comorbidities (bladder stones, diverticula, neoplasms, etc.), intravesical prostate protrusion, and prostate volume and shape. Prostate volume can be estimated from suprapubic approach with sufficient accuracy. The advantage of transrectal versus suprapubic ultrasound (TRUS) imaging is the possibility of evaluating prostate morphology and transitional zone index (TZI) which has been associated with a greater severity of LUTS in Korean men [1, 30].

Transrectal imaging of the prostate cannot be used to diagnose or rule out prostate cancer in patients with LUTS, but it should be used to guide accurate needle placement during transrectal prostatic biopsy or to allow accurate evaluation of prostate volume and gland morphology [29].

Currently, prostate ultrasound (transrectal or transabdominal) is considered as optional test in the specialized management of patients with LUTS/BPO. However, it may be an appropriate test when minimally invasive therapy or surgical operations are considered. The size and shape of the prostate and the presence of an intravesical lobe clearly evaluated by ultrasounds should be considered in selecting patients for transurethral microwave heat treatment (TUNA) or other minimally invasive therapy as well as for the selection of transurethral prostatic incision (TUIP) versus transurethral prostatic resection (TURP) [1].

Three-dimension ultrasonography, magnetic resonance imaging, and computer tomographic images are alternative method for lower urinary tract imaging with somewhat greater precision than transrectal or transabdominal ultrasonography, but their higher cost and lower availability of machines limit their usefulness in the routine assessment of patients with LUTS/BPO in the clinical setting [1, 30].

Bladder and Detrusor Wall Thickness

Although PFS is considered the standard method to diagnose BPO, several noninvasive tests have been tested in the last decades to overcome the invasiveness and costs associated with PFS. Bladder wall hypertrophy is evaluated by means of bladder wall thickness (BWT) and detrusor wall thickness (DWT), depending if the ultrasound calipers may in fact include only the muscular layer (DWT) or include the bladder mucosa and/or the adventitia (BWT), which have been recently investigated as alternatively noninvasive tests to predict the presence of BPO. The notion that the urinary bladder becomes "corrugated" and "thick in its coats" dates back to Avicenna and John Hunter, although whether detrusor hypertrophy is a natural effect of ageing or it reflects conditions that often occur in the elderly remains unclear [31].

Tubaro and Miano first proposed the analogy between the effects of an increased workload in the bladder and in the heart in 2002 [32]. Notwithstanding the obvious differences between the detrusor and heart muscle fibers at both levels increase, outlet resistance may develop in case of bladder outlet obstruction and arterial hypertension, respectively, leading to an early hypertrophy compensatory response, ultimately followed by decompensation leading to acute urinary retention and congestive heart failure, respectively. In cardiology, ultrasonography is standard of care to evaluate the hypertensive damage. In urology, suprapubic ultrasound of the urinary bladder has been applied only in the pediatric age.

In 1998, Manieri [14] and co-workers investigated the relationship between BWT and BOO. BWT was measured at 150 mm bladder-filling volume by a 3.5 MHz mechanical sector probe by different investigator blinded to patient voiding status. A threshold of 5 mm for BWT was identified for the diagnosis of BOO. Patients with BWT less than 5 mm were unobstructed in 63 % of cases at a pressure flow study while 88 % of those with BWT of 5 mm or greater were in the obstructed group according to the urethral resistance algorithm parameter. Analysis of the prognostic value of BWT for the diagnosis of BOO by the ROC analysis showed a higher prognostic index for BWT compared to peak flow rate with values under curve of 0.860 for BWT and 0.688 for peak flow rate. BWT was also able to distinguish between unobstructed cases in class 0 and I and the equivocal cases in class II and obstructed cases in class III or IV.

Further insights about measurement of BWT were provided more recently by Oelke and co-workers [21, 22] who evaluated the change of thickness values at various bladder volumes. Ultrasound evaluation of BWT was performed at the anterior bladder wall using a 7.5 MHz linear array positioned suprapubically in horizontal direction. The digital picture was enlarged to a factor 9.8 and detrusor wall was measured at least at three different sites. BWT continuously changed during the first 50 % of bladder capacity, while constant values of BWT were observed between 60 and 100 % of bladder capacity [21]. Recently, they also demonstrated that BWT is dependent on the bladder filling but only at a bladder-filling volume less than 250 ml. Oelke et al. [21] also obtained similar results. They evaluated BWT in 70 patients with LUTS. Mean detrusor wall thicknesses for unobstructed, equivocal, and obstructed patients were 1.33 mm (95 % CI, 1.17–1.48), 1.62 mm (95 % CI, 1.48–1.76), and 2.4 mm (95 % CI, 2.12–2.68). Differences were significant ($p<0.001$) between unobstructed and obstructed patients as well as between equivocal and obstructed patients. No significant difference was detected between nonobstructed and equivocal patients ($p=0.349$). A 2 mm threshold for BWT was considered as the best value for the diagnosis of BOO with the highest specificity (97.3 %) and positive predictive value (95.5 %) when compared to peak flow rate (25 and 55 %), residual urine (43.2 and 55.3 %), and prostatic volume (25 and 55.9 %). ROC analysis confirmed, as reported by Manieri and co-workers [4], that BWT is the best parameter to detect BOO with the highest area under the curve (AUC, 0.882) when compared to peak flow rate (AUC, 0.779), residual urine (AUC, 0.699), and prostate volume (AUC, 0.626). Subsequent studies have investigated the change in DWT before and after surgical treatment of BPO and they clearly showed that detrusor hypertrophy is significantly reduced by the relief of BPO [22, 28]. One year postoperatively, BWT was significantly reduced by 44.2 % after prostatic surgery (from 5.2 ± 0.7 to 2.9 ± 0.9 mm) and 93 % of patients were considered unobstructed according to the ICS nomogram. Decrease of BWT was evident 1 week after surgery (from 5.2 ± 0.7 to 3.3 ± 0.7 mm), reached a nadir at 6 weeks, and seems to remain stable up to 52 weeks. Although ultrasound evaluation of BWT or DWT appears quite promising, and recent attempts have been made to standardize the technique, its routine use is still limited. At present, measurement of BWT/DWT remains a promising research issue with a controversial use in clinical practice unless recently available automated ultrasound systems foster their clinical use.

In order to standardize the technology for the measurement of BWT/DWT, a dedicated instrument has been recently developed: the BladderScan BVM 6500 (Diagnostic Ultrasound, Bothell, WA). The instrument employs state-of-the-art technology for the measurement of bladder volume (24 isocentric scans of the bladder) and a special algorithm for automatic pattern recognition which identifies the other and inner borders of the bladder wall. Variability below 5 % was reported for bladder volumes of 200–400 ml [29]. Future studies should demonstrate that its routine clinical use can overcome the limitation associated with the manual ultrasound evaluation of bladder wall hypertrophy parameters.

Urodynamic

Urodynamics includes different tests although cystometry and pressure–flow study (PFS) are the most frequently performed ones. They have the unique capacity to diagnose BPO, detrusor overactivity, and detrusor underactivity which are considered to be associated with unfavorable outcome following TURP [29]. Furthermore, if simultaneous imaging is done (video-urodynamics), the site of BOO can be localized accurately at the bladder neck, the prostate, or the urethra. In addition, cystometry provides useful information regarding the function of the lower urinary tract during both the storage and voiding phases of the bladder cycle and in many instances can support a definitive pathophysiological diagnosis for the patient's LUTS [19]. Although different nomograms exist to assess BOO status, the International Continence Society nomogram together with the bladder outlet obstruction index (BOOI = detrusor pressure at $Q_{max} - 2Q_{max}$) should be used as the method of choice to define patients as obstructed, nonobstructed, or equivocal. Detrusor contractility strength during voiding can be also judged by different nomograms or can be obtained by calculating the bladder contractility index (detrusor pressure at maximum flow + $5Q_{max}$), also known as project isometric pressure (PIP) [1].

The rationale for using pressure–flow studies in the evaluation of men with LUTS related to BPH derives from the lack of correlation between symptoms, an enlarged prostatic gland, and the presence of BOO. Another important application for urodynamic test is prognosis and prediction of the outcome of treatment. Although no consensus has been reached yet as to the relation between BPO and the outcome of surgery, there is also a clear evidence in literature that the outcome of surgery is significantly better in men with obstruction than in those who are not obstructed as defined by preoperative pressure–flow studies and that urodynamic studies provide great predictive value of clinical improvement after prostatic relief but they also properly predict the poor clinical results in nonobstructed patients [30].

In patients with acute urinary retention, urodynamic studies are also useful in predicting the surgical outcome. Absence of detrusor overactivity, inability to void during PFS, and a maximum detrusor pressure <20 cmH$_2$O are associated with a poor outcome after surgery [1].

Although PFS is considered the standard method for the evaluation and grading of BOO and detrusor contractility, it is considered an additional optional test by several guidelines in the diagnostic work-up of patients with LUTS/BPO [30]. PFS must be considered an invasive procedure with possible side effects which make its routine clinical use still debated. Some authors also considered that the costs and invasiveness of PFS were not justified by the clinical advantages obtained [11, 16].

The NICE, the AUA guidelines, and the 6th International Consultation on New Developments in Prostate Cancer and Prostatic diseases completely agree that pressure–flow study remains the only means of establishing or ruling the presence of BOO and that patients considering surgery should have a definitive diagnosis of outlet obstruction, or if PFS is not planned prior to invasive treatment, then the patient should be aware of the diagnostic accuracy and limitation of uroflowmetry [1, 18]. The NICE recommendations also suggest that although PFS is considered an invasive test with associated costs, the information it provides is important to reduce unnecessary surgery and to possibly save associated costs [19]. PFS is also considered mandatory in the research setting to increase statistical power and reduce the number of patients at risk from novel treatments for BPO [1, 18, 19]. The EAU guidelines mostly agree with the other international guidelines and urodynamic studies are considered optional tests usually indicated in counseling patients before surgical treatment. In particular, they should be considered for patients prior to surgical treatment if they are young (<50 years) or elderly (>80 years); present high post-void residual (PVR>300 ml), a $Q_{max} \geq 15$ ml/s, neurogenic disorders, a previous radical pelvic surgery, or previous unsuccessful invasive treatment; or have bilateral hydronephrosis or cannot void more than 150 ml [20].

Endoscopy of the Lower Urinary Tract

Urethrocystoscopy is the standard endoscopic procedure to evaluate lower urinary tract. It can provide information about prostate length and bladder neck morphology and identify presence of bladder diverticula, trabeculation, or stones and of urethral stones, stenosis, or diverticula. Although the routine use of flexible instruments has reduced the invasiveness and discomfort associated with the procedure, routinely performed on outpatient basis, it presents a low diagnostic accuracy for the detection of BPO and remains optional in the specialized management of patients with LUTS/BPO in all the available guidelines or algorithms [1, 19, 30]. However, it should be appropriate in men with a history of recurrent UTI, sterile pyuria, microscopic or gross hematuria, urethral stricture, bladder cancer, prior lower urinary tract surgery, severe symptoms, or pain [1, 19, 30]. It is not recommended in patients on watchful waiting or medical therapy and it has been proposed as an optional test to identify whether surgery or another form of invasive therapy was suitable in men with severe LUTS [1].

Algorithms

In the last two decades, several national and international guidelines have been proposed for the management of patients suffering from LUTS/BPO. The ideal guidelines should be based on evidence medicine and expert opinion and should be very clear to address the right path to be followed by general practitioner or specialized physicians to correctly manage patients with LUTS/BPO. Most of the guidelines also developed diagnostic and therapeutic algorithms as a practical guide to better identify the proposed common work-up pathway to be initiated for a correct diagnosis and treatment of patients with LUTS/BPO.

The 6th International Consultation on New Developments in Prostate Cancer and Prostatic Diseases released a volume entitled *Male Lower Urinary Tract Dysfunction: Evaluation and Management*, with the intent to produce a modern approach incorporating both basic (family physicians and internists) and specialized (urologists) evaluation algorithms, and treatment strategies, driven by presenting symptoms [1, 26]. The guidelines suggest diagnostic tests, either a basic (Fig. 3.1) evaluation or a specialized evaluation depending on the severity of LUTS resulting from BPH (Fig. 3.2); it also identify recommended test to be done on every patient during the

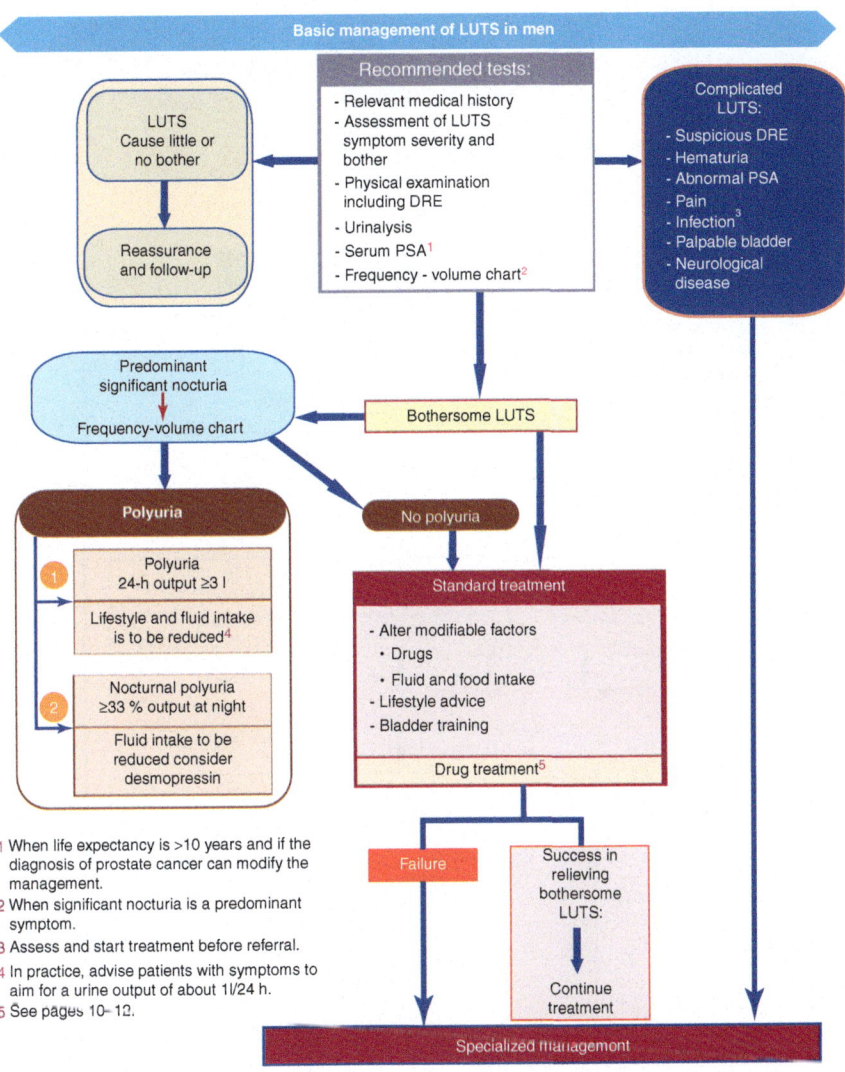

Fig. 3.1 Basic management of patients with LUTS according to the 6th Consultation on New Developments of Prostate Cancer and Prostatic Diseases (From McConnell et al. [17], with permission)

initial evaluation and an optional test to be considered in the evaluation of selected patients. In general, optional tests are done during a specialized evaluation, usually performed by urologists and which includes imaging of the prostate by transabdominal ultrasonography or TRUS, imaging of the upper urinary tract by ultrasonography or IVU, and endoscopy of the lower urinary tract and pressure–flow studies [1, 12].

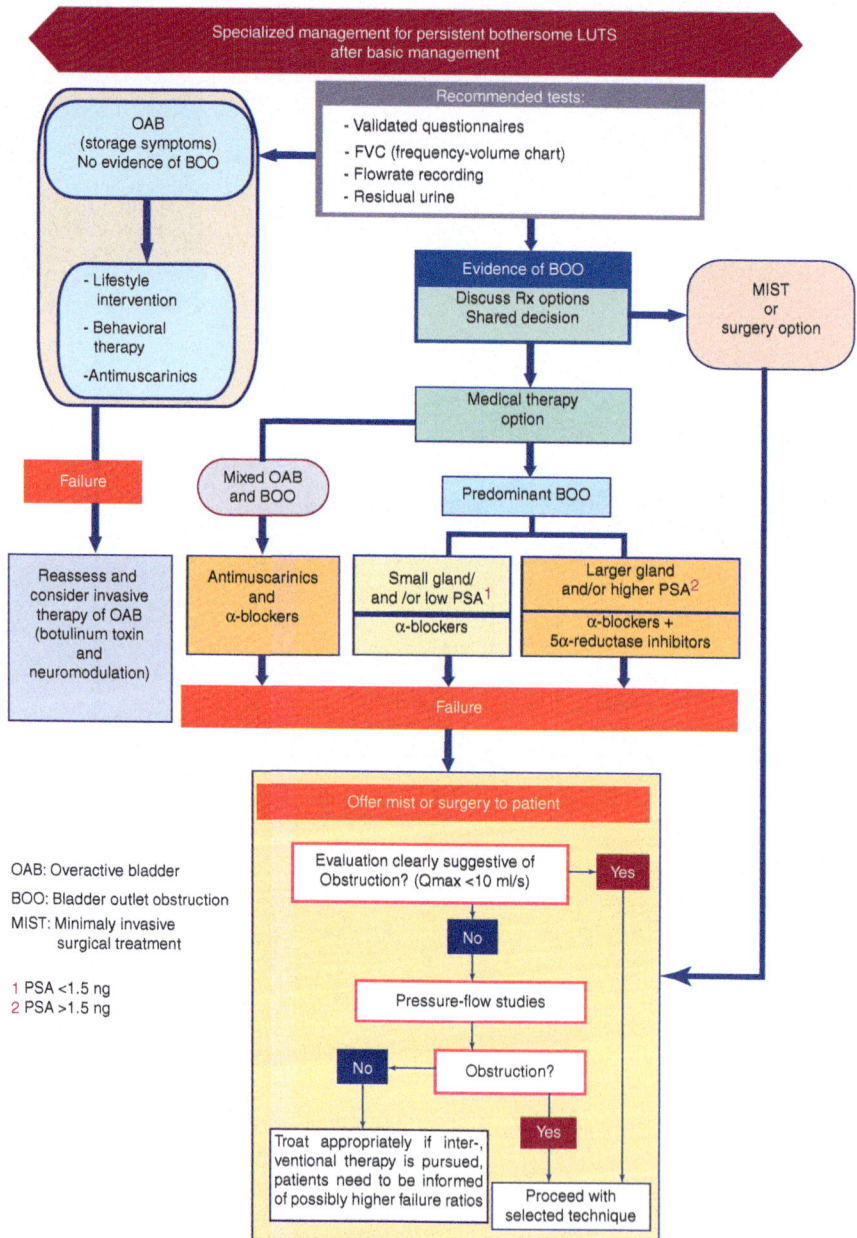

Fig. 3.2 Specialized management of patients with LUTS according to the 6th Consultation on New Developments of Prostate Cancer and Prostatic Diseases (From McConnell et al. [17], with permission)

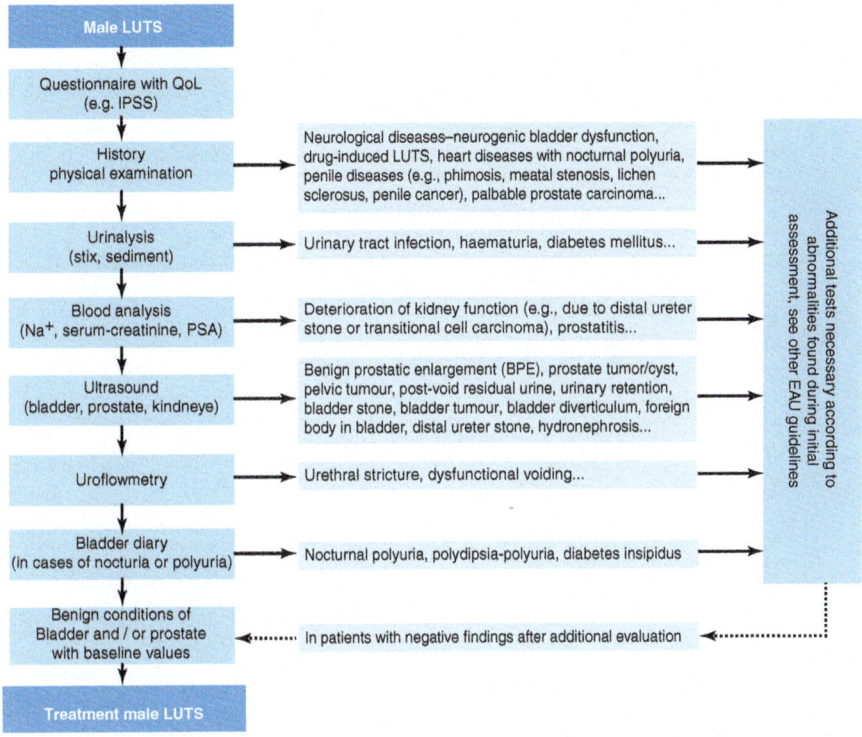

Fig. 3.3 Specialized management of patients with LUTS according to the European Association of Urology guidelines on management of LUTS (From Oelke et al with permission)

The AUA panel considered that the recommendations for diagnosis published by the 2005 International Consultation on Urologic Diseases are valid and do not deserve further study because they reflected a best practice in this area [10, 18].

In 2012, the EAU guidelines on management of male urinary tract symptoms including benign prostatic hyperplasia presented its own algorithms for the assessment of LUTS in men aged 40 years or older (Fig. 3.3). The algorithms proposed by the EAU are primarily intended to be used by urologist but can be used by general practitioners, and the proposed systematic work-up should exclude relevant diseases or conditions also causing LUTS in adult men. When relevant pathologies have been identified, the assessment may be interrupted [20].

The NICE [19] recently proposed a new guideline that covers men (18 and over) with a clinical working diagnosis of LUTS. The associated diagnostic algorithm firstly guides the physician in a diagnostic work-up to identify and correctly manage in patients with LUTS the occurrence of acute or chronic urinary retention and the presence of prostate cancer and of complicated or bothersome LUTS (Fig. 3.4).

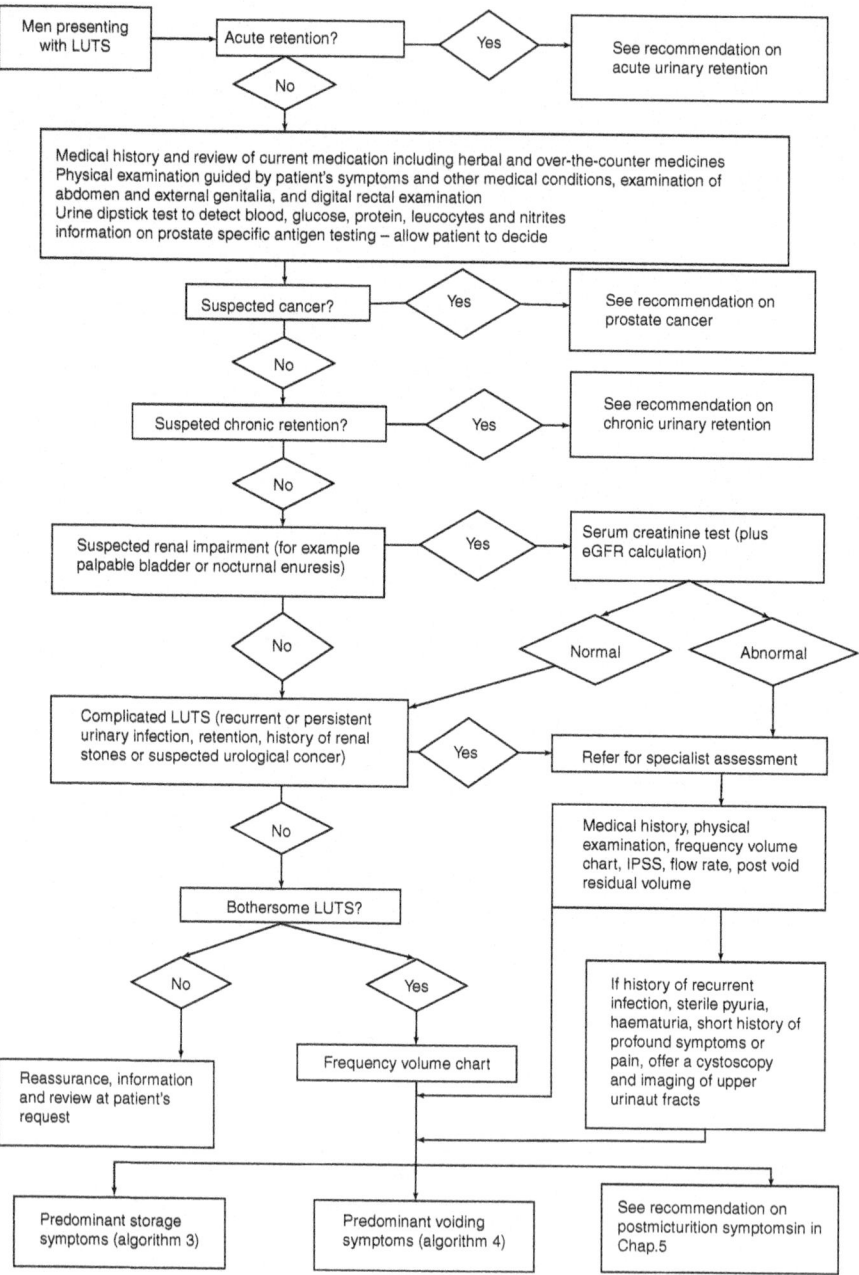

Fig. 3.4 Specialized management of patients with LUTS according to the National Clinical Guideline Centre (NICE) (From the NICE [19] CG 97, with permission)

Conclusion

In the last decade, the pathogenesis of LUTS/BPO has been completely investigated and revisited with significant implications on patient management. Recently, the 6th International Consultation on New Developments in Prostate Cancer and Prostatic Diseases, sponsored by the International Union against cancer (UICC), summarized the current understanding of the disease and outlined the definition of recommended and optional diagnostic tests that should be used in the assessment of patients with LUTS/BPO [1].

Recommended tests, to be performed in all patients with LUTS and BPE, included:

- Medical history
- Quantification of symptoms and bother
- Physical examination
- Urinalysis
- Biochemical tests
- Frequency–volume chart

Optional tests were considered:

- Uroflowmetry
- Post-void residual volume (PVR)
- Urinary tract imaging
- Pressure–flow studies
- Endoscopy of the lower urinary tract

However, there is no yet a consensus on how to properly and cost-effectively diagnose and treat patients with LUTS/BPO. The implementation and validation of the available algorithms proposed by the most important international urological association could improve patients' management, improve patients/physician communication, and ultimately avoid the number of unnecessary examinations in patients with LUTS/BPO and reduce the social costs of the disease.

References

1. Abrams P, D'ANcona C, Griffiths D, et al. Lower urinary tract symptom: etiology, patient assessment and predicting outcome from therapy. In: McConnell JD, Abrams P, Denis L, Khoury S, Roehrborn CG, eds. 6th International Consultation on New Developments in Prostate Cancer and Prostate Diseases, 2005. Paris, France: Health Publications; 2006: 71–141.
2. Abrams P, Chapple C, Khoury S, et al. Evaluation and treatment of lower urinary tract symptoms in older men. J Urol. 2009;181:1779.
3. Barry MJ, Fowler Jr FJ, O'Leary MP, Bruskewitz RC, Holtgrewe HL, Mebust WK, Cocket AT. The American Urological Association symptom index for benign prostatic hyperplasia. The Measurement Committee of the American Urological Association. J Urol. 1992;148(5): 1549–57.

4. Chapple CR, Roehrborn CG. A shifted paradigm for the further understanding, evaluation and treatment of lower urinary tract symptoms in men: focus on the bladder. Eur Urol. 2006;49(4):651–8.
5. Chodak GW, Kotler P, Shoenberg H. Routine screening for prostate cancer using the digital rectal examination. Prog Clin Biol Res. 1988;269:87.
6. Coyne K, Lai JS, Zyczynski T, et al. Validation of an overactive bladder awareness tool for use in primary care settings. Adv Ther. 2005;22(4):381–4.
7. Coyne K, Matza LS, Thomson C, et al. The responsiveness of the OAB-q among OAB patients subgroup. Neurourol Urodyn. 2007;26(2):196–203.
8. De Nunzio C, Aroson W, Freedland SJ, Giovannucci E, Kellog Parsons J. The correlation between metabolic syndrome and prostatic diseases. Eur Urol. 2012;61:560–70.
9. Griffiths D, Hofner K, van Mastrigt R, et al. Standardization of terminology of lower urinary tract function: pressure flow studies of voiding urethral resistance and urethral obstruction. Neurourol Urodyn. 1997;16:1–18.
10. Juliao AA, Plata M, Kazzazi A, Bostanci Y, Djavan B. American Urological Association and European Association of Urology guidelines in the management of benign prostatic hypertrophy: revisited. Curr Opin Urol. 2012;22:34–9.
11. Keqin Z, Zhishun X, Jing Z, et al. Clinical significance of intravesical prostatic protrusion in patients with benign prostatic enlargement. Urology. 2007;70(6):1096.
12. Kirby MG, Wagg A, Cardozo L, et al. Overactive bladder: is there a link to the metabolic syndrome in men? Neurourol Urodyn. 2010;29(8):1360–4.
13. Kupelian V, McVary KT, Kaplan SA, et al. Association of lower urinary tract symptoms and the metabolic syndrome: results from the Boston Area Community Health Survey. J Urol. 2009;182(2):616–24.
14. Manieri C, Carter S, Romano G, Trucchi A, Valenti M, Tubaro A. The diagnosis of bladder outlet obstruction in men by ultrasound measurement of bladder wall thickness. J Urol. 1998;159(3):761–5.
15. Mc Connel J, Roehrborn C, Bautista OM, et al. The long term effects of doxazosin, finasteride and combination therapy on the clinical progression of benign prostatic hyperplasia. N Engl J Med. 2003;349:2387–98.
16. McConnel JD. Why pressure-flow studies should be optional and not mandatory for evaluating men with benign prostatic hyperplasia. Urology. 1994;44:156.
17. McConnell JD, Abrams P, Khoury S, et al. Evaluation and treatment of lower urinary tract symptoms (LUTS) in older men. In: McConnell JD, Abrams P, Denis L, Khoury S, Roehrborn CG, eds. 6th International Consultation on New Developments in Prostate Cancer and Prostate Diseases, 2005. Paris, France: Health Publications; 2006:387–401.
18. McVary KT, Roehrborn CG, Avins AL, et al. Update on AUA guideline on the management of benign prostatic hyperplasia. J Urol. 2011;185:1793–803.
19. National Institute for Health and Clinical Excellence. CG 97 lower urinary tract symptoms: the management of lower urinary tract symptoms in men. London: NICE; 2010. Available from: www.nice.org.uk/guidance/CG97.
20. Oelke M, Bachmann A, Descazeaud A, et al. Guidelines on management of male lower urinary tract symptoms (LUTS) including benign prostatic obstruction. 2012. Available at: http://www.uroweb.org/fileadmin/user_upload/Guidelines/TreatmentofNonneurogenicmaleLUTS.pdf.
21. Oelke M, Hofner K, Grunewald BV, Jonas U. Increase in detrusor wall thickness indicates bladder outlet obstruction (BOO) in men. World J Urol. 2002;19:443–52.
22. Oelke M, Kirschner-Hermanns R, Thiruchelvam N, Heesakkers J. Can we identify men who will have complications from benign prostatic obstruction (BPO)? ICI-RS 2011. Neurourol Urodyn. 2012;31:322–6.
23. Resnick M, Ackermann R, Bosch J, et al. Initial evaluation of LUTS. In: Chatelain C, Denis L, Foo KT, et al., editors. Benign prostatic hyperplasia. Paris/Plymouth: Health Publication Ltd.; 2001. p. 169–202.

24. Roehrborn CG, Malice M, Cook TJ, Girman CJ. Clinical predictors of spontaneous acute urinary retention in men with LUTS and clinical BPH: a comprehensive analysis of the pooled placebo groups of several large clinical trials. Urology. 2001;58:210.
25. Roehrborn CG, Sech S, Montoya J, Rhodes T, Girman CJ. Interexaminer reliability and validity of three dimensional model to asses prostate volume by digital rectal examination. Urology. 2001;57:1087.
26. Roherborn CG. Currently available treatment guidelines for men with lower urinary tract symptoms. BJU Int. 2008;102 Suppl 2:18–23.
27. Staskin D, Kelleher C, Avery K, et al. Initial assessment of urinary and faecal incontinence in adult male and female patients. In: Abrams P, Cardoso L, Khoury S, Wein A, editors. Incontinence. Paris: Health Publication; 2009. p. 331–412.
28. Tubaro A, Carter S, Hind A, Vicentini C, Miano L. A prospective study of the safety and efficacy of suprapubic transvesical prostatectomy in patients with benign prostatic hyperplasia. J Urol. 2001;166(1):172–6.
29. Tubaro A, De Nunzio C. Benign prostatic hyperplasia. In: Chapple CCR, Steers WD, editors. Practical urology: essential principles and practice. London: Springer; 2011. p. 361–70.
30. Tubaro A, De Nunzio C, Trucchi A. Lower urinary tract symptoms suggestive of benign prostatic hyperplasia: what is the evidence for rational diagnosis? In: Muir G, Dawson C, editors. Evidence in urology, vol. 11. Bramhills; 2005. p. 89–96.
31. Tubaro A, Mariani S, De Nunzio C, Miano R. Bladder weight and detrusor thickness as parameters of progression of benign prostatic hyperplasia. Curr Opin Urol. 2010;20:37–42.
32. Tubaro A, Miano L. Managing the consequence of obstruction. Eur Urol. 2002;1(Suppl):21–7.

Chapter 4
Treatment Algorithms: When to Treat and Whom?

Nikesh Thiruchelvam

Abstract Over the last decade or so, a number of key international organizations have filtered the large body of emerging evidence examining the treatment of men with LUTS. This chapter distils these treatment guidelines starting with the most recent first. Most management algorithms divide treatment into conservative, medical, and surgical. There is also focus on acute and chronic urinary retention and nocturia. Fortunately, there is reasonable overlap signalling sound evidence and advice.

Keywords Algorithm • Conservative • Medical • Surgical • BPH • LUTS • Retention • Nocturia

Introduction

A number of treatment algorithms exist for the treatment of men with lower urinary tract symptoms. Men present to healthcare professionals because they have bothersome symptoms, they have developed or are concerned of developing acute urinary retention, or because of concerns of prostate cancer. The natural history of BPH outlined in earlier chapters shows that the risk of acute urinary retention is low, in the region of 3 % of men with moderate or severe bothersome LUTS. To date there is no correlation with specific LUTS and prostate cancer but clearly, such concerns need to be addressed in symptomatic men who present; relevant discussions and counselling about PSA and prostate biopsy will be often be required. These natural history studies also show an improvement or resolution of symptoms in around 30 % of men with LUTS. As such, a large number of men with symptomatic LUTS can be and should be assessed, diagnosed, and treated in primary care before onward referral to

N. Thiruchelvam
Department of Urology, Addenbrookes Hospital, Cambridge University Hospitals NHS Trust, Hills Road, Cambridge, CB2 0QQ, UK
e-mail: nikesh.thiruchelvam@addenbrookes.nhs.uk

urologists. In an aid to treat these patients and to standardize this "shared care," a number of treatment guidelines have been devised. They help the caregiver distinguish LUTS and BPH from other diseases with similar symptoms, determine disease severity, and risk of progression. They help in deciding on the best standard of care without undertaking the difficult task of being aware of the best available evidence [1]. There is emerging evidence to show that there is a large variation in practice in delivering BPH care by doctors [2] and also by urologists [3]. Adherence to guidelines results in greater use of medical therapy [4] and a lower reliance on surgery [5]. Guidelines have also been shown to improve confidence of primary care physicians and reduce secondary referrals and costs. This chapter describes these English language guidelines in greater detail and has been described in order of most recent.

European Association of Urology Guidelines [6]

At the time of going to press, these are the most current guidelines (see Fig. 4.1) and are based on a structured literature search by a guideline panel. The guidelines are primarily written for urologists. These guidelines describe in simple terms the recommended schedule for men presenting with lower urinary tract symptoms.

For those men with mild to moderate uncomplicated LUTS or who are not too bothered by their symptoms, they should be offered watchful waiting. This consists of education about the cause of their symptoms with reassurance that they do not have cancer. These points have been shown to improve symptoms and quality of life [7]. Lifestyle advice should also be given. This should include (based on consensus):

- Reduction of fluid intake
- Avoidance of caffeine and alcohol
- Double voiding
- Urethral milking for post-micturition dribble
- Bladder retraining (encouraged to "hold on" when they have urgency and to increase the time between voids)
- Treatment of constipation

Men with moderate to severe symptoms should be managed with an alpha-blocker. If the prostate volume is greater than 40 mls or PSA >1.4, a 5a-reductase inhibitor should be considered. If men have moderate to severe LUTS which are predominantly storage symptoms, muscarinic receptor antagonists should be offered but caution is needed in those with bladder outflow obstruction.

In those that have failed medical therapy or out of patient choice, surgery should be offered. Methods of BPO surgery are listed below based on prostate size. Again this remains a consensus view rather than due to high-quality evidence:

- TUIP/BNI for PV <30 mls
- TURP (monopolar or bipolar) or laser vaporization of the prostate for PV 30–80 mls
- Open prostatectomy or HoLEP for PV >80 mls

Minimally invasive options (TUMT, intraprostatic ethanol, prostatic stents) and newer laser modalities are considered experimental as the evidence base remains lacking.

NICE Guidelines on Male Lower Urinary Tracts Symptoms (2010) [8]

The National Institute of Clinical Health and Excellence published their guidance in 2010. The title reflects that men suffer from lower urinary tract symptoms and not just benign symptoms from prostatic enlargement. The guidance is based on the best available evidence following expert evaluation and consensus. The guideline development group consisted of four urologists, two GPs, a geriatrician, and representatives of patients and nurses. There is also a further guideline review panel that consists of members from the following perspectives: primary care, secondary care, lay, public health, and industry. This panel overseas development and ensures all registered stakeholders views are addressed.

Conservative and Drug Treatment (Figs. 4.1 and 4.2)

Men with storage LUTS should be offered advice on supervised bladder training, fluid intake, lifestyle advice and, if needed, containment products. Men with post-prostatectomy incontinence should be offered supervised pelvic floor muscle training. Urethral milking may help men with post-micturition dribbling. It may be reasonable to offer long-term urinary catheterization in men where medical treatment has failed and where surgery is not appropriate. Men with moderate to severe voiding LUTS should be offered an alpha-blocker and those with OAB symptoms should be offered an anticholinergic agent. In men with bothersome moderate to severe LUTS and prostates estimated to be larger than 30 g or a PSA level greater than 1.4 ng/ml, a 5-alpha-reductase inhibitor or a combination of an alpha-blocker and a 5-alpha-reductase inhibitor should be taken. In men with mild or moderate bothersome LUTS or those that fail drug therapy, reassurance maybe sufficient.

Surgery

If offering surgery, men should be offered TURP, TUVP, or HoLEP. Men with smaller prostates (<30 g) should be offered transurethral incision of the prostate. Open prostatectomy should be offered to men with prostates >80 g only. Minimally invasive treatments (TUNA, TUMT, HIFU, TEAP, and laser coagulation) should not be offered.

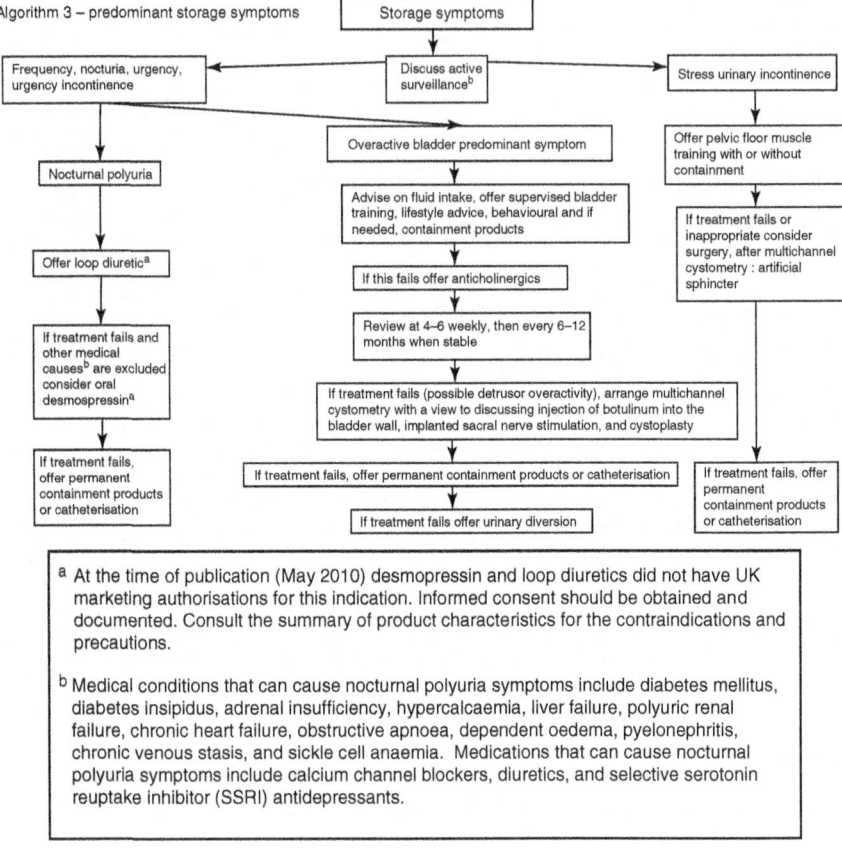

Fig. 4.1 Treatment of men with predominantly storage lower urinary tract symptoms (Accurate at the time of press: from Algorithm 3 Page 32, with permission)

Canadian Urology Association (2010): Guidelines for the Management of Benign Prostatic Hyperplasia [9]

This guideline recommends management based on literature published between 2000 and 2009. Guidelines are divided into diagnostic guidelines (further subdivided into mandatory, recommended, optional, or not recommended tests) and guidelines for treatment (which are standard of care, optional, or not recommended treatments).

Treatment

Standard care should be offered to men with mild symptoms, this should consist of lifestyle modifications and watchful waiting. The former may consist of:
- Fluid restriction
- Avoidance of caffeinated beverages and spicy foods

4 Treatment Algorithms: When to Treat and Whom?

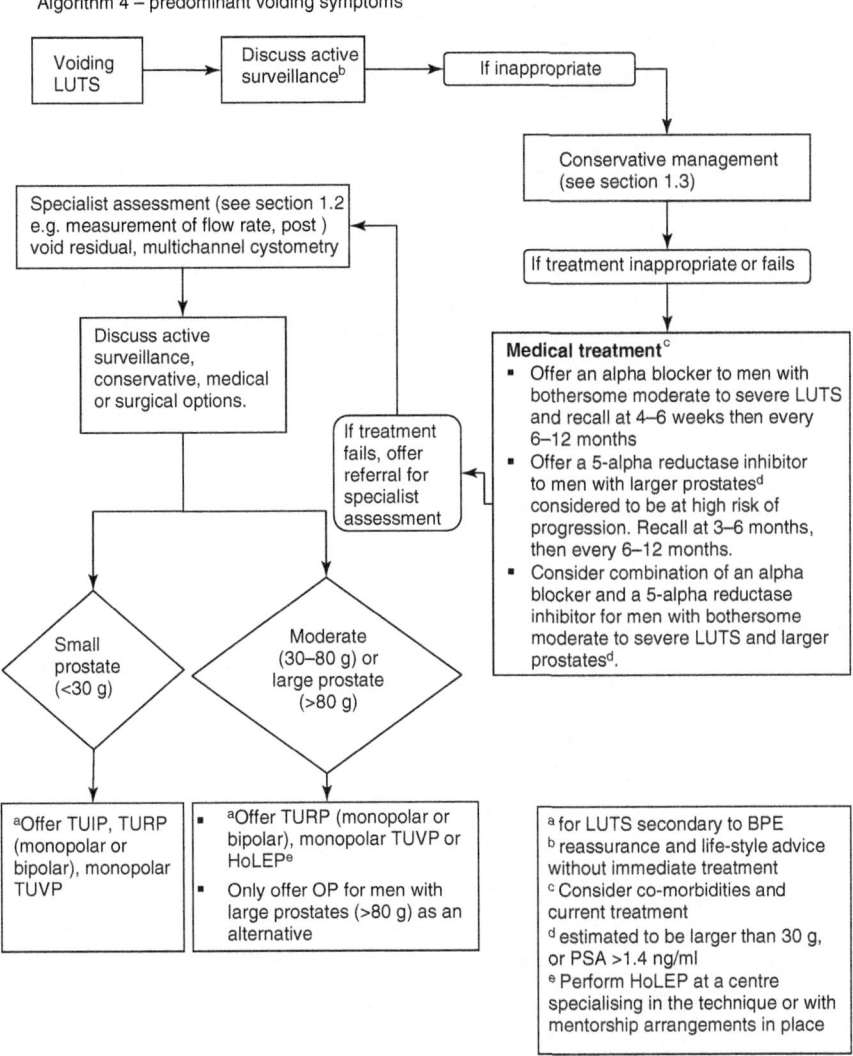

Fig. 4.2 Treatment of men with predominantly storage lower urinary tract symptoms (Accurate at the time of press: from Algorithm 4 Page 34, with permission)

- Avoidance/monitoring of some drugs (e.g., diuretics)
- Bladder retraining
- Pelvic floor exercises
- Avoidance or treatment of constipation

In addition to above, men with moderate to severe symptoms should be offered medical therapy and surgery. Optional medical treatment includes alpha-blockers, 5-alpha-reductase inhibitors or a combination of the two. Phytotherapy and phosphodiesterase inhibitors are not recommended in this guideline. Monopolar TURP is described as the gold standard surgical option with all forms of laser prostatectomy as acceptable alternatives. Further optional surgery includes TUIP for smaller prostates and open prostatectomy for larger prostates. TUNA, TUMT, and prostatic stents are acceptable optional treatments but absolute ethanol injection, HIFU, water-induced thermotherapy, and intraprostatic botulinum toxin injection are not recommended.

This guideline also has a special considerations section. It describes controversial optional treatments in the following groups:

- Symptomatic prostatic enlargement but without bothersome symptoms: men can be offered, after appropriate counselling, a 5-alpha-reductase inhibitor
- BPH-related bleeding: after ruling out worrying causes, consider a 5-alpha-reductase inhibitor or a TURP if persistent
- BPH and prostate cancer concern: if the patient has an elevated PSA and a negative prostate biopsy, consider a 5-alpha-reductase inhibitor for prostate cancer risk reduction

American Urological Association Guideline on the Management of BPH (2010) [10]

This guideline was published as an update to the 2003 guideline and was devised in a similar manner to previous publications – by expert review of the literature. Guidelines are listed as standard, recommended, and optional. This guideline outlines the shift in focus of treatment not just to alleviate bothersome LUTS but also focuses on altering disease progression and prevention of complications associated with BPH and LUTS. This guideline also highlights diseases linked to LUTS. This includes erectile dysfunction and lifestyle factors such as exercise, weight gain, and obesity.

The standard on treatment is that information on the benefits and harms of treatment alternatives for LUTS secondary to BPH should be explained to patients with moderate to severe symptoms (AUA-SI score ≥ 8) who are bothered enough to consider therapy and that patients with mild symptoms of LUTS secondary to BPH (IPSS <8) and patients with moderate or severe symptoms (IPSS ≥ 8) who are not bothered by their LUTS should be managed with watchful waiting. The guideline recognizes that levels of distress that individual patients are able to tolerate is highly variable so watchful waiting may be a patient's treatment of choice even if he they have a high IPSS score.

Conservative and Drug Treatment

Watchful waiting should include yearly review with DRE and/or serum PSA. Medical therapy includes alpha-blockers although the less prostate-selective agents (e.g., phenoxybenzamine) are not recommended. 5-ARIs may be used in combination with alpha-blockers and also in isolation to prevent progression of LUTS. No specific values are outlined but combination therapy is appropriate for men with demonstrable prostatic enlargement based on prostate volume, PSA level (as a proxy for volume), and/or enlargement on DRE. 5-ARIs are also recommended for the treatment of refractory hematuria but not to reduce intraoperative bleeding prior to a TURP. In recognition that LUTS may be due to OAB, anticholinergic agents are recommended but are to be used with caution in men with a PVR >250 mls. Dietary supplement and phytotherapeutic agents are not recommended.

Surgery

In addition to the usual transurethral and laser resection and enucleation techniques, TUMT and TUNA are also described as potential options for surgical treatment. Open prostatectomy is also an option but there is insufficient evidence to recommend laparoscopic and robotic prostatectomy. This guideline states that the choice of approach should be based on the patient's presentation, anatomy, the surgeon's level of training and experience, and a discussion of the potential benefit and risks for complications. The presence of a bladder diverticulum is not an absolute indication for surgery unless associated with recurrent UTI or progressive bladder dysfunction.

International Consultation on Urological Diseases (2006): Male Lower Urinary Tract Dysfunction [11]

This is a very detailed evidence-based document that attempts to ignore or downplay guidelines based on expert opinion rather than evidence.

Alpha-blockers are first-line drug therapy for BPO and failure of treatment appears to occur in one-fifth of patients. Causes of failure include insufficient efficacy, development of acute urinary retention, and adverse events associated with the medication [12] and is associated with increasing age, higher IPSS, and larger prostate volume. This consultation outlines that TURP is the gold standard surgical treatment for BPO and given that TURP is expensive and does not always lead to symptom improvement, predictors of success such as unequivocal obstruction and normal detrusor contractility should be identified. Due to lack of evidence, this document does not attempt to identify a treatment algorithm but does identify future areas of research.

Management of Benign Prostatic Hyperplasia: South African Urological Association Guideline (2006) [13]

This pharma-sponsored consensus document outlines investigation and management as the above but also lists drugs to be avoided in patients with BPH. These included testosterone (known to cause prostate enlargement and growth), alpha-adrenergic agonists (e.g., ephedrine, may cause bladder neck contraction), anticholinergic agents (e.g., antispasmodics and antiparkinsonian agents, may impair detrusor contraction), and diuretics (may cause frequency and nocturia).

Guideline for the Primary Care Management of Male Lower Urinary Tract Symptoms (2004) [14]

This guideline was developed following a literature review by the authors, representing the British Association of Urology, and is at aimed specifically at GPs, nurse practitioners, and patients. The document outlines primary care assessment in keeping with the above guidelines but with some minor changes. Assessment tests have been divided into recommended (history and examination and urinalysis), optional (frequency-volume chart, serum creatinine, PSA, post-void residual measurement, flow rate, and urodynamics), and not recommended (renal tract ultrasound, transrectal ultrasound, and cystoscopy).

Acute Urinary Retention

The International Continence Society defines AUR as a painful, palpable, or percussible bladder when the patient is unable to pass any urine. However, AUR is not always painful (e.g., after regional anesthesia). Patients are typically catheterized and then undergo a trial without catheter while taking an α-blocker which is known to improve the success of trial without catheter after AUR. This was first demonstrated with alfuzosin [15] and then later with tamsulosin. In the former ALFAUR study, 62 % passed their TWOC after alfuzosin as compared to nearly 50 % of men who successfully passed their TWOC after 3 days of placebo. A successful TWOC with an α-blocker also reduces the chance of needing future prostate surgery. If the trial of voiding fails, the patient should be considered for surgical intervention. Prostate size is thought to possibly predict the chance of a successful TWOC and also for the need for future surgery. Urodynamics is also a useful predictor of successful improvement in LUTS voiding after a TURP in patients with AUR. Old age, absence of detrusor overactivity, inability to void during the voiding phase, and a low maximum detrusor pressure are predictors of poor outcome after a TURP. If a patient presents in AUR while already on an α-blocker, and they have no precipitating causes (e.g., UTI, constipation), surgery on the bladder outlet is now commonly performed.

Chronic Urinary Retention

The International Continence Society defines chronic urinary retention as a nonpainful bladder, which remains palpable or percussible after the patient has passed urine. It is typically associated with a residual volume (RV); there is no consensus as to what defines a RV but many would regard >300 mls as a significant RV but this number will depend on a number of ill-defined factors such as age and detrusor contraction. NICE defines CUR as >1,000 mls. Another problem is that there is marked intraindividual variation when measuring PVR. Similarly, a palpable bladder may not diagnose CUR. Using a cutoff of 25 cm H_2O bladder end filling pressure and a PVR of 300 mls, CUR has been defined at urodynamics as high pressure (HPCR) and low pressure (LPCR) [16]. It is more common to have renal deterioration and upper urinary tract dilatation with HPCR. These men may also present with nocturnal enuresis. These patients need urgent catheterization and then a subsequent surgery to relieve obstruction, long-term catheterization or learn to perform clean intermittent self-catheterization (CISC) (Fig. 4.3). These men should not undergo a TWOC without undergoing one of these procedures or very close surveillance. In men with LPCR, men are likely to have better symptom control with surgery or CISC. In the elderly age group with LPCR, possibly over the age of 80, men are likely to not do well in the long term with any sort of surgery [17].

Nocturia and Nocturnal Polyuria

Nocturia is the complaint that the individual has to wake at night (or during times of normal sleep) one or more times to void. Each void should be preceded and followed by sleep. It should be considered part of the normal aging process with an increasing incidence from the age of 50. Nocturia affects 55 % of men over 70 and 70–90 % of men over 80. Nocturia is present with equal incidence in both men and women.

The cause of nocturia is multifactorial with each of the following also having many causes:

- Sleep disorder – with age, sleep time and efficiency decreases and there is increased frequency of awakenings and sleep apnea
- Nocturnal polyuria – defined as >20–33 % of the total urine production occurs at night (depending on the patient age). This could be considered normal physiology – the proportion of urine production at night increases in the elderly (up to 50 % of total urine production). Potential causes include a) venous fluid redistribution (from venous insufficiency and/or congestive heart failure) when changing to the recumbent position at night and b) an abnormality in the secretion and/or action of arginine vasopressin at night
- Polyuria from habitual excess fluid intake, diabetes mellitus (glucose-induced osmotic diuresis), and diabetes insipidus (impaired excretion of AVP or insensitivity to AVP). Polyuria is defined as approximately greater than 40 ml per kg body weight per 24 h
- BPO and DO – results in reduced voided volumes and increased micturition frequency as a result of reduced bladder capacity

In addition to history and examination, the frequency-volume chart will be essential in diagnosing nocturia, possible nocturnal polyuria, and continuous

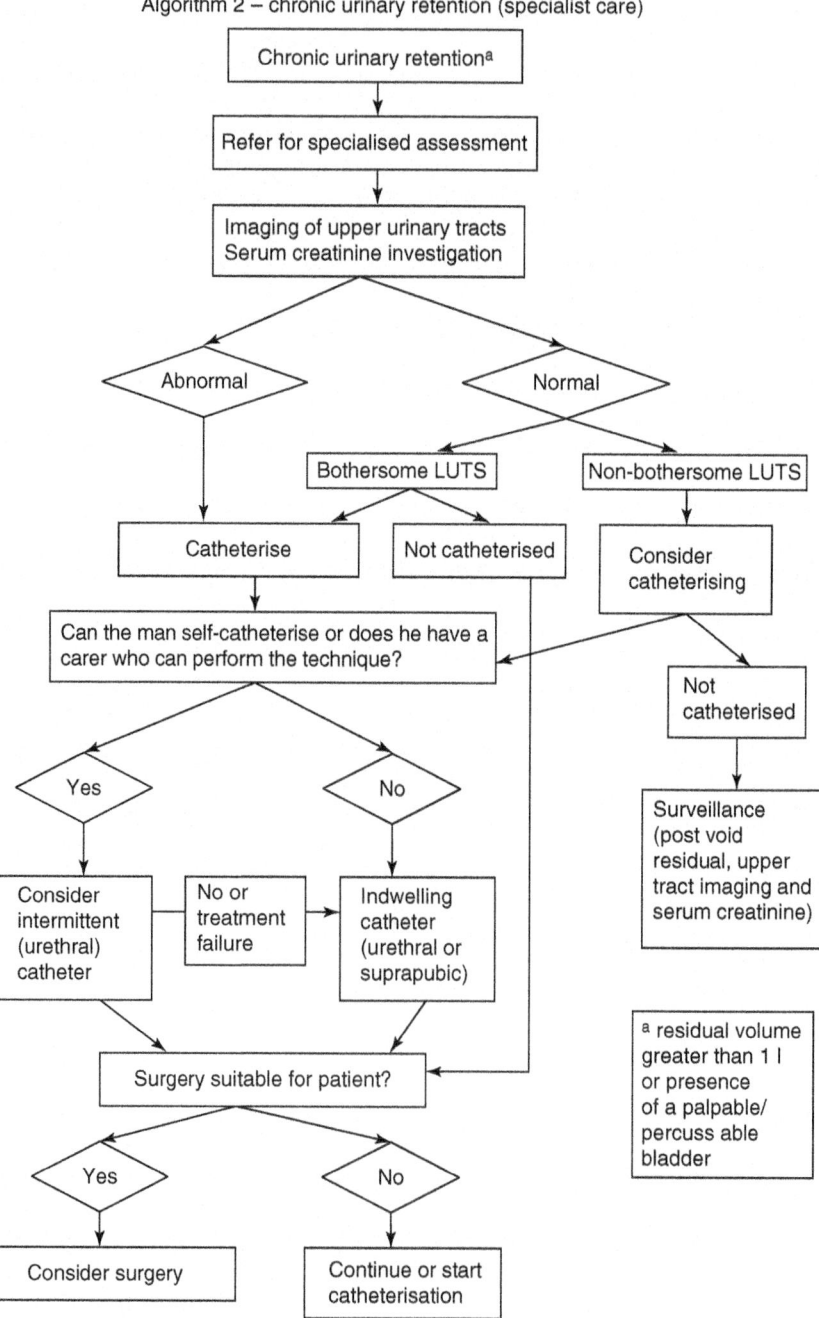

Fig. 4.3 Treatment Algorithm for chronic urinary retention (specialist care) (Accurate at the time of press: from Algorithm 2 Page 31, with permission)

polyuria. Treatment involves conservative therapy and drug therapy but this field remains under-researched. Measures include:

- Stopping oral fluid intake beyond 7 p.m.
- Elevating the legs during the day when sedentary
- Treatment of any sleep disorder, e.g., with positive pressure ventilation for sleep apnea
- A loop diuretic in the early afternoon (to promote voiding of volume overload in the evening rather than at night)
- Antimuscarinic therapy if DO is a main contributing factor
- Exogenous AVP (desmopressin or DDAVP) to replace the reduced excretion of AVP in the elderly at night. Strict review of serum electrolytes is necessary if a patient is started on this because of the risk of fluid retention and dilutional hyponatremia

Conclusions

When good evidence is available, there are many similarities in published guidelines. Variability occurs when the evidence is less robust. There are also minor variations in international and country-specific guidelines. Guidelines can be lengthy, expensive, and time consuming; one of the first guidelines, US Guidelines on BPH by the Agency for Health Care Policy and Research (AHCPR), published in 1994, took 3 years to complete. Guidelines encourage standardized treatment and promote improved care. All the above treatment algorithms are in agreement that men with bothersome LUTS should seek and be offered treatment.

References

1. Juliao AA, Plata M, Kazzazi A, Bostanci Y, Djavan B. American Urological Association and European Association of Urology guidelines in the management of benign prostatic hypertrophy: revisited. Curr Opin Urol. 2012;22(1):34–9. Epub 2011/11/30.
2. Emberton M. Medical treatment of benign prostatic hyperplasia: physician and patient preferences and satisfaction. Int J Clin Pract. 2010;64(10):1425–35. Epub 2010/06/29.
3. Strope SA, Elliott SP, Saigal CS, Smith A, Wilt TJ, Wei JT. Urologist compliance with AUA best practice guidelines for benign prostatic hyperplasia in Medicare population. Urology. 2011;78(1):3–9. Epub 2011/05/24.
4. Norg RJ, van de Beek K, Portegijs PJ, van Schayck CP, Knottnerus JA. The effectiveness of a treatment protocol for male lower urinary tract symptoms in general practice: a practical randomised controlled trial. Br J Gen Pract. 2006;56(533):938–44. Epub 2006/11/30.
5. Strope SA, Wei JT, Smith A, Wilt TJ, Saigal CS, Elliott SP. Evaluative care guideline compliance is associated with provision of benign prostatic hyperplasia surgery. Urology. 2012;80(1):84–9. Epub 2012/05/23.
6. Oelke M, Bachmann A, Descazeaud A, Emberton M, Gravas S, Michel MC, et al. EAU guidelines on the treatment and follow-up of non-neurogenic male lower urinary tract symptoms including benign prostatic obstruction. Eur Urol. 2013;64(1):118–40. Epub 2013/03/13.

7. Brown CT, Yap T, Cromwell DA, Rixon L, Steed L, Mulligan K, et al. Self management for men with lower urinary tract symptoms: randomised controlled trial. BMJ. 2007;334(7583):25. Epub 2006/11/23.
8. National Institute for Health and Care Excellence. The management of lower urinary tract symptoms in men. CG 97. 2010. London: National Institute for Health and Care Excellence.
9. Nickel JC, Mendez-Probst CE, Whelan TF, Paterson RF, Razvi H. 2010 update: guidelines for the management of benign prostatic hyperplasia. Can Urol Assoc J. 2010;4(5):310–6. Epub 2010/10/15.
10. McVary KT, Roehrborn CG, Avins AL, Barry MJ, Bruskewitz RC, Donnell RF, et al. Update on AUA guideline on the management of benign prostatic hyperplasia. J Urol. 2011;185(5): 1793–803. Epub 2011/03/21.
11. Mcconnell Pa J, Denis L, Khoury Cr S. Male lower urinary tract dysfunction. Paris: Health Publications; 2006.
12. Hong SJ, Ko WJ, Kim SI, Chung BH. Identification of baseline clinical factors which predict medical treatment failure of benign prostatic hyperplasia: an observational cohort study. Eur Urol. 2003;44(1):94–9; discussion 99–100. Epub 2003/06/20.
13. Bereczky Z, Bolus M, Chetty P, du Toit W, Enslin J, Haffejee M, et al. Management of benign prostatic hyperplasia – South African Urological Association Guideline. S Afr Med J. 2006;96(12 Pt 3):1275–9. Epub 2007/01/26.
14. Speakman MJ, Kirby RS, Joyce A, Abrams P, Pocock R. Guideline for the primary care management of male lower urinary tract symptoms. BJU Int. 2004;93(7):985–90. Epub 2004/05/15.
15. McNeill SA, Hargreave TB, Roehrborn CG. Alfuzosin 10 mg once daily in the management of acute urinary retention: results of a double-blind placebo-controlled study. Urology. 2005;65(1):83–9; discussion 89–90. Epub 2005/01/26.
16. Abrams PH, Dunn M, George N. Urodynamic findings in chronic retention of urine and their relevance to results of surgery. Br Med J. 1978;2(6147):1258–60. Epub 1978/11/04.
17. Thomas AW, Cannon A, Bartlett E, Ellis-Jones J, Abrams P. The natural history of lower urinary tract dysfunction in men: minimum 10-year urodynamic follow-up of untreated detrusor underactivity. BJU Int. 2005;96(9):1295–300. Epub 2005/11/17.

Chapter 5
Medical Treatment of LUTS/BPH

Giacomo Novara, Vincenzo Ficarra, and Filiberto Zattoni

Abstract Several drug therapies are available for male patients with bothersome lower urinary tract symptoms. Monotherapy with α-blockers is a commonly used and effective treatment to quickly improve LUTS, quality of life, and Q_{max}. The main differences among the drugs are in the profile of adverse events [AEs], with cardiovascular AEs less prevalent with uroselective drugs (and especially with the novel silodosin, which is the compound with the highest selectivity). Conversely, ejaculatory dysfunction is less prevalent with nonselective drugs. 5α-reductase inhibitors [5-ARIs], alone or in combination with α-blockers, might be offered to men who have moderate to severe LUTS and an enlarged prostate to reduce the risk of urinary retention and prostate-related surgery. Those patients with prevalent storage LUTS may have benefited from anticholinergics. The risk of urinary retention with that category of drugs is minimal if patients with a higher risk of bladder outlet obstruction are avoided (e.g., those with PVR >200 mL, Q_{max} <5 mL/s, or history of prior retention). Finally, tadalafil 5 mg is effective in improving symptoms in patients with LUTS, with or without concomitant erectile dysfunction.

Keywords BPH • LUTS • α-Blockers • 5α-Reductase inhibitors • Anticholinergic drugs • Phosphodiesterase type 5 inhibitors • Alfuzosin • Tamsulosin • Silodosin • Finasteride • Dutasteride • Tadalafil

---

G. Novara (✉) • V. Ficarra • F. Zattoni
Department of Oncological and Surgical Sciences,
Urology Clinic, University of Padua, Via Giustiniani 2, Padua 35100, Italy
e-mail: giacomonovara@gmail.com, giacomo.novara@unipd.it

Introduction

The international guidelines available for the treatment of male lower urinary tract symptoms (LUTS) suggestive of benign prostatic hyperplasia (BPH) identify accurately those patients who need treatment for their symptoms [1–3]. All patients with bothersome LUTS are usually regarded as candidates for treatment, as well as those patients with complicated LUTS (e.g., patients with recurrent urinary tract infections [UTIs], acute or chronic urinary retention, bladder stones). In patients with uncomplicated LUTS, treatment is triggered by the impairment of a patient's quality of life, regardless of LUTS severity. Consequently, patients with bothersome mild LUTS (i.e., American Urological Association Symptom Index [AUA-SI] <8) may be considered for treatment, whereas patients with moderate LUTS (i.e., AUA-SI 8–18) or, rarely, severe LUTS (i.e., AUA-SI >18) who are not bothered by the symptoms may not need treatment.

The purpose of treatment is usually twofold. Therapy has to improve symptoms as quickly as possible, reducing LUTS severity as well as their impact on quality of life in those patients with uncomplicated LUTS. For patients with complicated LUTS, treatments must also aim at resolving complications (e.g., allowing catheter removal in patients with acute urinary retention [AUR]). More recently, such a symptomatic approach has been coupled with an increasing interest in a long-term preventive approach, with the goal of reducing the risks of worsening symptoms, the occurrence of complications, or eventual surgery.

In patients with uncomplicated LUTS, patient preference usually dictates the choice among the various medical and surgical treatments. Although uncommon in clinical practice, patients may elect to skip medical treatments and select surgical therapy to achieve faster and more significant improvement of their LUTS. However, most patients with uncomplicated LUTS elect to try medical therapies as first-line treatment.

Options for Nonsurgical Treatment of Lower Urinary Tract Symptoms

The simplest treatment for LUTS patients is modifications of lifestyle [1, 2]. These include reduction in fluid intake, avoidance/moderation of alcohol and caffeine intake, bladder retraining, and using timed voiding schedules. All these measures are simple and inexpensive tools that have been shown to be very effective in improving LUTS. Brown et al. randomized 140 patients to lifestyle modifications plus standard treatment (represented by watchful waiting) vs. standard treatment alone. The primary outcome was treatment failure, defined as an increase of three or more points on the International Prostate Symptom Score (IPSS), use of drugs to control LUTS, AUR, or surgical intervention during follow-up. Treatment failure was significantly more common in the control arm at 3-month follow-up (difference between arms 32 %; $P<0.0001$), 6-month follow-up (difference 42 %; $P<0.0001$), and 12-month follow-up (difference 48 %; $P<0.0001$). Patients randomized to self-management had significant improvements in IPSS at 3-month follow-up (IPSS differences between the 2 arms: 5.7 points; $P<0.0001$), 6-month follow-up (difference: 6.5 points; $P<0.0001$), and 12-month follow-up (difference: 5.1 points; $P<0.0001$) [4].

In addition, whenever possible, discontinuation of drugs that may aggravate bladder outlet obstruction or may affect lower urinary tract function (e.g., tricyclic antidepressants or diuretics) and treatment of constipation should always be attempted.

In cases where these nonpharmacologic therapies are not sufficiently effective, several categories of drugs are available on the market including α-blockers (mainly doxazosin, terazosin, tamsulosin, and, more recently, silodosin), 5α-reductase inhibitors [5-ARIs] (finasteride and dutasteride), anticholinergics (mainly oxybutynin, tolterodine, solifenacin, and fesoterodine), phytotherapies (mainly *Serenoa repens* and other saw palmetto extracts), or a combination. A recent population-based study evaluating BPH-related drugs prescribed in 19 European countries from 2004 to 2008 demonstrated that α-blockers (alone or in association with other drugs) are the most widely prescribed drugs, accounting for about 70 % of the yearly 11.6 million prescriptions, whereas 5-ARIs represents about 20 % of them, although the 5-ARI share of the market is slowly increasing. Plant extracts accounted for about 17 % of the market, although prescription rates across European countries vary widely [5].

Very recently, tadalafil, a phosphodiesterase type 5 inhibitor [PDE5-I], well known for its use in erectile dysfunction [ED] patients, was approved by both the US Food and Drug Administration [FDA] and the European Medicines Agency [EMA] for the treatment of men with LUTS, with or without concomitant ED, providing a new drug for treatment of male LUTS.

α-Blockers

α-Blockers affect the action of endogen catecholamines on prostate stromal smooth muscle, where $α_{1A}$ receptors are present, reducing the smooth muscle tone and extent of obstruction [1]. However, it has been hypothesized that endogen catecholamines may also act on different subtypes of $α_1$-receptors (i.e., $α_{1B}$ and $α_{1D}$) present in other areas of the lower urinary tract, in the spinal cord, or in blood vessels.

Alfuzosin, doxazosin, and terazosin are usually considered nonselective drugs, inhibiting all the different $α_1$-receptor subtypes. Conversely, tamsulosin and, above all, silodosin have higher selectivity for $α_{1A}$ receptors [6]. All the α-blockers available on the market for several years (alfuzosin, doxazosin, tamsulosin, and terazosin) have been extensively studied, and although head-to-head comparative studies are rare, they are currently regarded as equally clinically effective drugs in improving patient symptoms (IPSS improvement of about 35–40 %), patient quality of life due to LUTS, and maximum flow rate (Q_{max}; Q_{max} improvements of 20–25 %), as demonstrated by systematic reviews performed by the Cochrane Collaboration and AUA guidelines panel [2, 7, 8].

However, major differences do exist in the adverse events (AEs) of the different drugs. Postural hypotension is more prevalent with nonselective α-blockers (prevalence rates close to 10 %). Conversely, ejaculatory dysfunction is more frequent with tamsulosin (prevalence of about 10 %) [2, 7, 8]. The literature available on silodosin, the most recent drug of the category, is more limited. However, the available randomized controlled trials [RCTs] suggest that silodosin reduces the IPSS score about 3 points more than placebo and improves Q_{max} about 1 mL/s more than placebo [9–11], whereas clinical efficacy compared with tamsulosin is similar [11].

A recent systematic review and meta-analysis of RCTs evaluating silodosin in the treatment of nonneurogenic LUTS demonstrated that silodosin was more effective than placebo with regard to mean change in IPSS total score (weighted mean difference [WMD] −2.62; $P<0.000001$), IPSS storage subscore (WMD −0.82; $P<0.000001$), IPSS voiding subscore (WMD −1.8; $P<0.000001$), IPSS quality-of-life item (WMD: −0.39; $P<0.0001$), and Q_{max} (WMD: 0.86; $P=0.0003$) [12].

Silodosin was more effective than tamsulosin 0.2 mg with regard to mean change in IPSS voiding subscore (WMD −0.75; $P=0.03$), IPSS quality-of-life item (WMD −0.26; $P=0.02$), and Q_{max} (WMD 0.71; $P=0.05$). Conversely, only a nonstatistically significant trend in favor of silodosin compared with tamsulosin 0.2 mg was found with regard to mean change in IPSS total score (WMD −1.48; $P=0.08$) and IPSS storage subscore (WMD −0.31; $P=<0.14$). Finally, silodosin and tamsulosin 0.4 mg were at least as effective in all the efficacy analyses [12].

With regard to AEs, the available RCTs demonstrated a high prevalence of ejaculatory dysfunction (ranging from 14 to 28 % in the different RCTs). However, other AEs, including cardiovascular AEs, were as prevalent in silodosin patients as with placebo [9–11], reconfirming the high uroselectivity of the drug. The systematic review just cited demonstrated that overall AEs (odds ratio [OR]: 2.05; $P=0.07$), ejaculatory dysfunction (OR: 33.4; $P<0.0001$), and withdrawal due to AEs (OR: 2.53; $P=0.001$) were all more common with silodosin than with placebo. Conversely, headache (OR: 1.22; $P=0.79$), dizziness (OR: 2.07; $P=0.07$), and AEs other than ejaculatory dysfunction (OR: 1.56; $P=0.48$) were similar with silodosin and placebo.

In comparison with tamsulosin, overall AE rates (OR: 1.54; $P=0.03$) and ejaculatory dysfunction (OR: 15.97; $P<0.00001$) were more prevalent with silodosin than with tamsulosin 0.2 mg. Conversely, AEs other than ejaculatory dysfunction were less prevalent with silodosin than with tamsulosin 0.2 mg (OR: 0.68; $P=0.03$), whereas withdrawal due to AEs was similar with the two drugs (OR: 0.79; $P=0.62$). With regard to the comparisons between silodosin 8 mg and tamsulosin 0.4 mg, ejaculatory dysfunction was less common with tamsulosin 0.4 mg (OR: 7.76; $P<0.00001$), whereas AEs other than ejaculatory dysfunction were more common with tamsulosin 0.4 mg (OR: 0.71; $P=0.05$). Finally, overall AEs (OR: 1.32; $P=0.08$), dizziness (OR: 1.25; $P=0.75$), and withdrawal due to AEs (OR: 2.04; $P=0.25$) were similar with silodosin 8 mg and tamsulosin 0.4 mg [12].

In conclusion, monotherapy with α-blockers is a commonly used and effective treatment to quickly improve LUTS, quality of life, and Q_{max}. The main differences among the drugs are in the profile of AEs, with cardiovascular AEs less prevalent with uroselective drugs (and especially with the novel silodosin, which is the compound with the highest selectivity). Conversely, ejaculatory dysfunction is less prevalent with nonselective drugs.

Monotherapy with 5α-Reductase Inhibitors and Combination Therapy with α-Blockers

5-ARIs decrease the conversion of testosterone to dihydrotestosterone, which is the more powerful metabolite. Finasteride inhibits subtype 2 of 5α-reductase, mainly present within the prostate, whereas dutasteride blocks both subtypes 1 and 2 of 5α-reductase.

Most of the available studies concern finasteride, which has been on the market for several years. Several RCTs showed that finasteride was significantly more efficacious than placebo both in treating LUTS and reducing prostate volume if prostate volume was larger than 30 cm^3 and therapy was continued for at least 6–12 months [13–16]. In the Finasteride Long-Term Efficacy and Safety Study, a large prospective RCT that enrolled more than 3,000 patients randomized to 4-year treatment with finasteride or placebo, McConnell et al. demonstrated IPSS improvements at the end of the study of 3.3 points in the finasteride arm and 1.3 points in the placebo arm (mean difference 2.1; 95 % confidence interval [CI], 2.6–1.6; $P<0.001$). Similarly, the mean increase in Q_{max} was 1.9 mL/s in the finasteride arm and 0.2 mL/s in the placebo arm (mean difference between groups 1.7 mL/s; 95 % CI, 1.3–2.1; $P<0.001$). Finally, an overall mean decrease in prostate volume of 18 % was observed in the finasteride arm as compared with an overall increase of 14 % in the placebo arm (mean difference 32 %; 95 % CI, 28–36; $P<0.001$) [17].

Similarly, Roehrborn et al. demonstrated that dutasteride was also more effective than placebo in reducing prostate volume (starting after 1 month of treatment) and improving both AUA-SI (starting after 6 months of treatment) and Q_{max} (starting as early as after 1 month of treatment) [18]. Roehrborn et al. reported on a total of 4,325 men with moderate to severe LUTS, Q_{max} 15 mL/s or less, prostate volume of 30 cm^3 or more at transrectal ultrasonography, and prostate-specific antigen (PSA) ranging from 1.5 to 10.0 ng/mL enrolled into three identical registrational RCTs and randomized to 24-month treatment with dutasteride 0.5 mg daily or placebo. After 24 months of treatment, AUA-SI improved 4.5±6.6 and 2.3±6.8 points in the dutasteride and placebo arms, respectively (mean difference 2.2 points; $P<0.001$); Q_{max} improved 2.2±5.2 and 0.6±4.7 mL/s in the dutasteride and placebo arms, respectively (mean difference 1.6 mL/s; $P<0.001$); finally, prostate volume decreased 14.6±13.5 cm^3 in the dutasteride arm, whereas it increased 0.8±14.3 cm^3 in the placebo arm (mean difference 15.4 cm^3; $P<0.001$) [18].

Both finasteride and dutasteride are usually well tolerated. However, AEs are not uncommon, especially sexual function. Loss of libido, ED, and ejaculatory dysfunction are present in about 5, 6, and 3 %, respectively, in patients taking finasteride according to a recent Cochrane meta-analysis [19]. Similarly, dutasteride is associated with risks of loss of libido, ED, and ejaculatory dysfunction in 4, 7, and 2 %, respectively [18].

To date, only a single randomized study has compared the 2 drugs head-to-head in the category. The Enlarged Prostate International Comparator (EPIC) study randomized about 1,600 men 50 years or older to receive a 12-month treatment with dutasteride 0.5 mg ($n=813$) or finasteride 5 mg ($n=817$). The primary end point was a change in prostate volume. The study failed to demonstrate any significant decrease in prostate volume between the two drugs. AUA-SI improvements, which were secondary study end points, were also similar in the two arms [20]. However, the study was underpowered to detect differences in IPSS changes. The 12-month treatment duration reported in the EPIC study is not the most appropriate time frame to assess treatment benefits of 5-ARIs, which are usually greater in longer-term treatment.

Other than symptom improvements, 5-ARIs can confer benefit in preventing disease progression. In 1998, the Finasteride Long-Term Efficacy and Safety Study demonstrated that finasteride over a 4-year period was able to reduce the risk of developing AUR (absolute risk reduction 4 %; relative risk reduction 57 %; $P<0.001$) and the need for surgery (absolute risk reduction 5 %; relative risk reduction 55 %; $P<0.001$) compared with placebo [17].

Due to the opportunity to prevent disease progression with long-term use of 5-ARIs as well as to obtain short-term improvement with α-blockers, combination therapies with the two categories of drugs have been widely tested.

In the Veterans Affairs Cooperative Benign Prostatic Hyperplasia Study, the first large RCT on combination therapy, 1,229 patients with moderate to severe LUTS, PSA less than 10 ng/mL, Q_{max} ranging from 4 to 15 mL/s, and no limits in prostate size were treated with terazosin, finasteride, placebo, or a combination for 12 months. Patients with the combination treatment showed a significant reduction in AUA-SI from baseline (−6.2 points), which was significantly higher than the reduction achieved by the 5-ARI monotherapy (−3.2) or placebo (−2.6) but not significantly different from terazosin monotherapy (−6.1). Q_{max} improvements also overlapped for combination therapy (+3.2 mL/s) and terazosin monotherapy (+2.7 mL/s) [20].

Similarly, the Alfuzosin-Finasteride study randomized 1,051 patients with LUTS to receive either alfuzosin or finasteride or a combination of both for 6 months, demonstrating that combination therapy was significantly more effective than finasteride monotherapy in reducing IPSS (6.1 vs. 5.2 points; $P=0.03$) but as effective as alfuzosin monotherapy (6.1 vs. 6.3) [21]. Similar results were also achieved in the Prospective European Doxazosin and Combination Therapy trial that compared 52-week treatments with doxazosin, finasteride, or a combination [22].

Significantly different conclusions were obtained in the Medical Therapy of Prostatic Symptoms (MTOPS) study, a large RCT that randomized more than

3,000 patients with moderate to severe LUTS and Q_{max} ranging from 4 to 15 mL/s to a 4.5-year treatment with finasteride 5 mg, doxazosin 8 mg, or their combination [23]. The primary end point of the study was clinical progression, defined as a four or more points worsening in AUA-SI, or the occurrence of AUR, UTIs, urinary incontinence, or renal function impairment. At follow-up, the study demonstrated a significant reduction in the risk of progression in patients treated with combination therapy as compared with placebo (risk of progression 1.5 per 100 person-years of follow-up in the combination therapy arm vs. 4.5 per 100 person-years of follow-up in the placebo arm; absolute risk reduction 3 %; relative risk reduction 66 %), finasteride monotherapy (risk of progression 2.9 per 100 person-years of follow-up), and doxazosin monotherapy (risk of progression 2.7 per 100 person-years of follow-up). The study reconfirmed that finasteride was able to prevent the occurrence of AUR as well as the need for LUTS surgery. However, combination therapy was as effective as finasteride monotherapy for the secondary end points [23].

In conclusion, the combination of finasteride and doxazosin was shown to be significantly more effective than monotherapies in reducing the overall risk of progression (which notably was represented only by AUA-SI worsening in about 60 % of the cases). However, in long-term treatment, finasteride monotherapy was as effective as combination therapy in reducing the risk of LUTS complications and surgical treatments.

Although MTOPS was clearly a positive study demonstrating the planned improvement in the primary end point with combination therapy, several clinical and methodological issues make the study conclusions more questionable. The overall risk of progression in the placebo arm was quite low (4.5 per 100 person-years of follow-up), and the absolute reduction in the risk of progression during combination therapy was also very low (about 3 per 100 person-years of follow-up). Consequently, the numbers needed to treat (i.e., the number of patients who have to be treated with combination therapy over 4.5 years to prevent a single event) was quite high (8 to prevent a single case of disease progression, 11 to prevent a single case of ≥4 points worsening AUA-SI, 51 to prevent a single case of AUR, and 29 to prevent a single case of LUTS surgery). Considering the relatively benign nature of the events we are hoping to prevent, the costs of long-term combination therapies, and the risk of treatment-related complications, it is clear that combination therapy cannot be considered an appropriate treatment for every patient, according to the MTOPS data. Several secondary analyses of MTOPS allowed us to identify patients with prostate volume more than 40 mL, PSA higher than 1.5 ng/mL, or Q_{max} less than 10 mL/s as those with a higher risk of progression [24, 25] where consequently combination therapy may achieve higher benefit and have a more favorable cost-effectiveness profile.

Further data on combination therapy were provided by the Combination of Avodart and Tamsulosin (CombAT) trial, another large RCT that assessed long-term combination therapy [26]. The study randomized more than 4,800 patients 50 years and older with a clinical diagnosis of BPH, IPSS 12 or higher, prostate volume 30 cm^3 or more, PSA ranging from 1.5 to 10 ng/mL, and Q_{max} more than 5 and

15 mL/s or less with minimum voided volume 125 mL or more to 4-year treatment with dutasteride monotherapy, tamsulosin monotherapy, or their combination.

The primary study end point at 2 years was the change in IPSS from baseline, whereas the 4-year primary end point was time to first AUR- or BPH-related surgery. Secondary end points at 4 years included BPH clinical progression, symptoms, Q_{max}, prostate volume, safety, and tolerability. With regard to IPSS modifications, the CombAT trial found that mean IPSS decrease from baseline to month 24 was 6.2 ± 0.15 points for combination therapy vs. 4.9 ± 0.15 and 4.3 ± 0.15 points for dutasteride and tamsulosin monotherapy, respectively. The IPSS decrease for combination therapy was significantly greater vs. that of either monotherapy (all P values <0.001). Such differences were statistically significant from month 3 for combination therapy vs. dutasteride and from month 9 for combination therapy vs. tamsulosin. With regard to AUR- or BPH-related surgery, combination therapy was significantly more effective in reducing the risk of such events as compared with tamsulosin monotherapy (absolute risk of AUR- or BPH-related surgery 4.2 % in the combination therapy arm vs. 11.9 % in the tamsulosin arm; absolute risk reduction 7.7 %; relative risk reduction 65.8 %; $P<0.001$).

Conversely, the differences between combination therapy and dutasteride monotherapy were not statistically significant (absolute risk of AUR- or BPH-related surgery 5.2 % in dutasteride arm; absolute risk reduction 1 %; relative risk reduction 65.8 %, $P=0.18$). Finally, combination therapy was more effective than either monotherapy in reducing the 4-year overall risk of BPH clinical progression, defined as more than a 4-point IPSS worsening and the occurrence of AUR, urinary incontinence, recurrent UTIs, or renal function impairment [26]. In summary, the CombAT study reconfirmed the advantages of combination therapy shown in the MTOP trial in a group of patients with a higher risk of progression, as suggested by older age, larger prostate volume, and higher PSA values.

Such advantages in the relief of symptoms and reduction of the risk of disease progression, however, come at the cost of a higher risk of treatment-related AEs. The MTOPS study found that dizziness (5.3 cases per 100 person-years of follow-up), postural hypotension (4.3 cases per 100 person-years of follow-up), ED (5.1 cases per 100 person-years of follow-up), abnormal ejaculation (3 cases per 100 person-years of follow-up), and decreased libido (2.5 cases per 100 person-years of follow-up) were all significantly more common with combination therapy than placebo. Moreover, 27, 24, and 18 % of the patients receiving doxazosin, finasteride, or combination therapy, respectively, discontinued drugs by the end of the study, mostly because of AEs [23].

Similarly, in the CombAT study, 28 % of the patients randomized to combination therapy experienced AEs (vs. 21 % in the dutasteride arm vs. 19 % in the tamsulosin arm; $P<0.001$), and 6 % of the patients discontinued drugs by the study end (vs. 4 % in the dutasteride arm vs. 4 % in the tamsulosin arm). The most prevalent AEs recorded in the CombAT trials were ED (9 % in the combination therapy arm vs. 7 % in the dutasteride arm vs. 5 % in the tamsulosin arm, respectively), loss of libido (4 % in the combination therapy arm vs. 3 % in the dutasteride arm vs. 2 % in the tamsulosin arm, respectively), and ejaculatory dysfunction

(4 % in the combination therapy arm vs. <1 % in the dutasteride arm vs. 1 % in the tamsulosin arm) [26].

In conclusion, 5-ARIs might be offered to men who have moderate to severe LUTS and an enlarged prostate to reduce the risk of AUR and future prostate-related surgery, as highlighted by both the European Association of Urology (EAU) and AUA guidelines [1, 2]. The National Health Service National Institute for Health and Clinical Excellence (NICE) guidelines recommend limiting the use of 5-ARIs in patients with LUTS who have prostates estimated to be larger than 30 g or a PSA level greater than 1.4 ng/mL who are considered at high risk of progression [3]. Similarly, combination therapy is suggested for men "with moderate to severe LUTS, enlarged prostates, and reduced Q_{max}" by the EAU guidelines [1], for men "with LUTS associated with demonstrable prostatic enlargement based on volume measurement, PSA level as a proxy for volume, and/or enlargement on digital rectal examination" by AUA guidelines [2], and for men "with bothersome moderate to severe LUTS and prostates estimated to be larger than 30 g or a PSA level greater than 1.4 ng/mL" by the NICE guidelines [3].

Anticholinergic Drugs

Anticholinergic drugs are commonly adopted in patients with overactive bladder [OAB] syndrome. They act as muscarinic receptors antagonists, blocking the acetylcholine action in detrusor smooth muscle cells, urothelial cells, and the peripheral or central nervous system [1]. Among the 5 muscarinic receptors subtypes (M1–M5) described in humans, M2 and M3 subtypes are those predominantly expressed in the urinary bladder and are supposed to be involved in detrusor contraction. The most commonly used anticholinergic drugs (darifenacin, fesoterodine, oxybutynin, solifenacin, tolterodine, and trospium) have been extensively studied in several RCTs and meta-analyses evaluating patients with OAB syndrome. They have been shown to reduce the number of urgency episodes and micturitions significantly compared with placebo [27].

Several studies evaluated the efficacy of such a category of drugs in patients with LUTS suggestive of BPH [27], based on the fact that about 50 % of those patients have storage symptoms. Kaplan et al. reported on more than 800 patients, 40 years or older, who had a total IPSS 12 or higher, IPSS quality-of-life item score 3 or higher, self-rated bladder condition of at least moderate bother, and a bladder diary documenting micturition frequency (8 or more micturitions per 24 h) and urgency (≥3 episodes per 24 h), with or without urgency urinary incontinence.

Those patients were randomized to a 3-month treatment with tamsulosin 0.4 mg, tolterodine extended release (ER) 4 mg, their combination, or placebo. Exclusion criteria were the presence of postvoid residual (PVR) volume more than 200 mL or Q_{max} less than 5 mL/s [28]. The primary efficacy end point was patient perception of treatment benefit at week 12, defined as answers to the questions "Have you had any benefit from your treatment?" and, if so, "Have you had little benefit or much benefit?"

After the 3-month treatment, 80 % of the patients randomized to combination therapy reported treatment benefit, as compared with 70 and 65 % of those receiving tamsulosin or tolterodine monotherapy, respectively, and 62 % of those randomized to placebo, with combination therapy more effective than either monotherapies (P values 0.03 vs. tamsulosin, 0.001 vs. tolterodine, and <0.001 vs. placebo).

Similarly, combination therapy was significantly more effective than monotherapies in improving overall daily number of micturitions, daily number of urgency episodes, total IPSS, and IPSS quality-of-life item score. The most prevalent AEs in the combination therapy arm was dry mouth (21 % vs. 7 % with either monotherapy or 2 % with placebo). Notably, only 2 patients (1 %) in the combination therapy arm as well as 4 (2 %) in the tolterodine arm, 4 (2 %) in the placebo arm, and 0 in the tamsulosin arm experienced AUR, demonstrating the low risk of AUR with anticholinergic drugs.

Further data are available from the Solifenacin and Tamsulosin in Males with Lower Urinary Tract Symptoms (SATURN) study, a phase 2 RCT that enrolled about 900 men with LUTS ($\geq$3 months, total IPSS $\geq$13, and maximum urinary flow rate 4.0–15.0 mL/s) [29]. Patients were randomized to a 12-week treatment with either tamsulosin oral controlled absorption system 0.4 mg; solifenacin 3, 6, or 9 mg; solifenacin 3, 6, or 9 mg plus tamsulosin; or placebo. The primary efficacy end point was change from baseline in total IPSS, whereas secondary end points included change from baseline to end of treatment in IPSS voiding and storage subscores, micturition diary variables (micturition frequency, urgency episodes of Patient Perception of Intensity of Urgency Scale grade 3 or 4, urgency incontinence episodes, and mean volume voided per micturition), and quality-of-life assessments (IPSS-QoL index and Patient Perception of Bladder Condition [PPBC]). The study failed to demonstrate any significant difference in IPSS improvements among tamsulosin and combination treatment arms. Conversely, decreases from baseline to end of treatment in micturition frequency and total urgency and frequency score and increases in voided volume per micturition were significantly greater with an increased solifenacin dose plus tamsulosin vs. tamsulosin monotherapy [29]. Also in the SATURN study, the combination therapy of α-blockers and anticholinergic drugs was well tolerated, with AEs in line with the known safety profiles of each individual drug.

More interesting from a practical point of view, some RCTs evaluated the efficacy of anticholinergic drugs as add-on therapy to patients treated with α-blockers with insufficient benefit. Chapple et al. reported on 652 men 40 years or older with frequency, urgency, and at least moderate problems reported on the PPBC, despite being on a stable dose of α-blockers for 1 month or longer [30]. Those patients were randomized to a 12-week treatment with tolterodine ER 4 mg daily or placebo while continuing their prescribed α-blocker therapy. The primary study end point was the percentage of subjects reporting improvement from baseline on the PPBC ($\geq$1 point) at week 12. Improvement in PPBC ratings was reported by 63.6 % of men receiving tolterodine ER plus α-blocker vs. 61.6 % of those randomized to placebo plus α-blocker ($P=0.66$). However, patients receiving tolterodine experienced significantly greater reductions in most of the bladder diary end points including 24-h micturitions (−1.8 vs. −1.2; $P=0.0079$); daytime micturitions (−1.3 vs. −0.8; $P=0.0123$); 24-h urgency episodes (−2.9 vs. −1.8; $P=0.0010$); daytime urgency episodes (−2.2 vs. −1.4; $P=0.0017$) and nocturnal urgency episodes (−0.5 vs. −0.3; $P=0.0378$); and frequency–urgency sum (−7.8 vs. −5.1; $P=0.0065$) as well as IPSS storage subscore (−2.6 vs. −2.1; $P=0.0370$) compared with placebo. However, AEs (mainly dry mouth, constipation, and headache) were significantly more prevalent in the patients receiving tolterodine (34.7 % vs. 27.6 %) [30].

Similar results were achieved in the VESicare in Combination with Tamsulosin study, a 12-week double-blind placebo-controlled trial assessing the safety and tolerability of solifenacin plus tamsulosin in men with residual OAB symptoms after tamsulosin monotherapy [31]. A total of 397 patients with a mean of 8 or more daily micturitions and 1 or more daily urgency episodes after taking 0.4 mg tamsulosin once daily for 4 or more weeks were randomized to a 12-week treatment with solifenacin 5 mg or placebo. The primary end point was mean change from baseline to week 12 in micturitions per 24 h, measured by a 3-day bladder diary. Secondary end points included changes from baseline to weeks 4, 8, and 12 in urgency, and, in scores on the PPBC, Urgency Perception Scale, and total IPSS. Solifenacin add-on therapy was not more effective than placebo in reducing the mean number of daily micturitions at week 12 (adjusted mean change −1.05 in the solifenacin arm vs. −0.67 in the placebo arm; treatment difference 0.38; $P=0.135$). However, daily urgency episodes were significantly lower in the solifenacin arm (adjusted mean change −2.18 in the solifenacin arm vs. −1.1 in the placebo arm; treatment difference 1.08; $P<0.001$) [31].

In conclusion, anticholinergics are an appropriate treatment for patients with prevalent storage symptoms, and the risk of AUR is minimal if patients with a higher risk of bladder outlet obstruction are avoided (e.g., those with PVR >200 mL, Q_{max} <5 mL/s, or history of prior AUR) [1–3]. Such drugs can be used in monotherapy in those patients with prevalent storage LUTS suggestive of OAB syndrome as well as in combination with α-blockers in those patients with persistent storage LUTS following α-blocker monotherapy.

Phytotherapy

Several plant extracts are currently used in the treatment of LUTS including *Serenoa repens*, *Pygeum africanum*, *Hypoxis rooperi*, *Urtica dioica*, *Secale cereale*, and *Cucurbita pepo*. *Serenoa repens*, the most commonly used preparation, is an n-hexane lipido/sterolic extract of the berry of the American dwarf palm tree and has antiandrogenic action and anti-inflammatory and antiproliferative pro-apoptotic effects [32]. A recent Cochrane meta-analysis demonstrated no advantage for *Serenoa repens* compared with placebo for relieving LUTS and improving Q_{max} [33].

These findings were corroborated by a recent large RCT evaluating almost 400 patients that also failed to demonstrate any efficacy of Prosta Urgenin Uno, a

Serenoa repens extract produced by Rottapharm/Madaus, over a period of 72 weeks, despite dose escalation up to 960 ng/day [34]. Based on such data, both EAU and AUA guidelines do not recommend the use of plant extracts in the treatment of male LUTS [1, 2].

Different producers use different extraction techniques, distribute active ingredients with different qualitative and quantitative properties, or combine 2 or more herbal compounds in one pill. The extracts of the same plant produced by different companies do not necessarily have the same biologic or clinical effects, so the effects of one brand cannot be extrapolated to others [35]. Even different batches of the same producer might contain different concentrations of active ingredients and cause different biologic effects [36]. Consequently, the pharmacokinetic properties can differ significantly between different plant extracts [1], and the literature results are difficult to interpret.

The literature is very limited on the combination of plant extracts and α-blockers [37, 38]. Glemain et al. randomized 352 men with IPSS 13 or higher and Q_{max} from 7 to 15 mL/s randomized to a 52-week treatment with tamsulosin 0.4 mg plus *Serenoa repens* 320 mg vs. tamsulosin 0.4 mg plus placebo. The study failed to demonstrate any statistically significant difference between combination therapy and tamsulosin monotherapy in IPSS total score improvements (−6.0 vs. −5.2, for combination and tamsulosin, respectively; $P=0.286$) and in all the other secondary end points [37]. Similar results were achieved in another small nonrandomized study including only 60 patients [38].

Phosphodiesterase Type 5 Inhibitors

PDE5-Is (sildenafil, tadalafil, and vardenafil) are the standard treatment for most patients with ED. Epidemiological data suggest that LUTS and ED are often co-prevalent diseases in adult men. The Multinational Survey of the Aging Male-7 survey demonstrated that about 50 % of the patients between 50 and 59 years of age with moderate to severe LUTS had concomitant ED, with those percentages even higher in patients between ages 60 and 69 and 70 and 79 years [39]. In such patients, most of the available drugs for LUTS may affect sexual function, whereas PDE5-Is might be a useful tool to treat both conditions with the same pill.

Mechanism of action of PDE5-Is in male LUTS is not completely clear. However, actions of PDE5-Is have been hypothesized on several pathways, including nitric oxide/cyclic guanosine monophosphate signaling, increased RhoA kinase activity, increased bladder afferent activity, and pelvic ischemia [40]. In vitro studies showed that sildenafil relaxes human prostate strips and inhibits the growth of prostatic smooth muscle cell [41], and sildenafil was shown to improve IPSS in open-label studies in ED patients [42]. Since that original report, several RCTs evaluating all PDE5-Is in LUTS patients have been reported [43, 44].

McVary et al. reported the first RCT evaluating PDE5-Is for LUTS in men with ED and LUTS [41]. A total of 370 men, 45 years or older, who scored 25 or less on the erectile function domain of the International Index of Erectile Function [IIEF] and 12 or more on IPSS were randomized to a daily dose of sildenafil 50 (each night at bedtime or 30 min to 1 h before sexual activity, with dose escalation to 100 mg after 2 weeks) or placebo. Finally, the RCT demonstrated that sildenafil was more effective than placebo in improving the overall score of the IPSS (−6.32 vs. −1.93; $P<0.0001$) and IPSS quality-of-life item score (−0.97 vs. −0.29; $P<0.0001$) in patients with concomitant ED and LUTS. Conversely, Q_{max} was not significantly modified (0.31 vs. 0.16; $P=0.8$) [41].

Subsequently, Stief et al. compared 8-week treatment with vardenafil 10 mg twice daily and placebo in patients with moderate to severe LUTS without ED, demonstrating a significant effect of vardenafil on the IPSS (−5.9 vs. −3.6; $P=0.0013$) [45]. However, due to differences in half-life (3.7 h of sildenafil vs. 3.3–3.9 of vardenafil vs. 17.5 h of tadalafil) [46], tadalafil is the most appealing drug in the PDE5-I family for LUTS treatment because a single dose may provide a 24-h long effect [47]. McVary et al. demonstrated in an RCT that 5 mg tadalafil for 6 weeks, followed by dose escalation to 20 mg for 6 weeks, was more effective than 12 weeks of placebo in improving IPSS (−7.1 vs. −4.5; $P<0.0001$) [48].

Roehrborn et al., in a large dose-finding RCT, randomized more than 1,000 men 45 years or older with a total IPSS 13 or higher and Q_{max} of 4–15 mL/s to a 12-week daily treatment with tadalafil 2.5, 5, 10, 20 mg or placebo. The primary study end point was the IPSS change after 12 weeks of treatment with 5 mg tadalafil compared with placebo. The study demonstrated that tadalafil 5 mg was significantly more effective than placebo in improving IPSS (−4.87 vs. −2.27 in the placebo arm; $P<0.001$), whereas the increases in IPSS with tadalafil 10 or 20 mg were only slightly better than with the 5-mg dose. AEs were more common with tadalafil 5 mg than with placebo (30.7 % vs. 21.2 %), with dyspepsia (4.7 %), and extremity pain (2.4 %) the most common [49].

Based on the data of the dose-finding study, Porst et al. reported a phase 3 RCT randomizing 325 men 45 years of age or older with BPH-LUTS for more than 6 months, IPSS 13 or higher, and a Q_{max} 4 or higher to 15 mL/s or less to 12-week treatment with tadalafil 5 mg or placebo [50]. The primary study end point was change in IPSS from baseline to week 12. At study end, tadalafil 5 mg was significantly more effective than placebo in improving overall IPSS (−5.6 vs. −3.6 in the placebo arm; $P=0.004$), as well as IPSS storage (−2.3 vs. −1.3 in the placebo arm; $P=0.002$), voiding (−3.3 vs. −2.3 in the placebo arm; $P=0.02$), and quality-of-life item (−1 vs. −0.7 in the placebo arm; $P=0.013$) scores. Notably, improvements in Q_{max} (1.6 vs. 1.1 in the placebo arm; $P=0.30$) and PVR volume (8.8 vs. 4.5 mL in the placebo arm; $P=0.50$) were not significantly different in the treatment and control arms. The proportion of subjects reporting AEs was similar between groups (26 % for tadalafil vs. 22 % for placebo), with headache (3.7 % vs. 0.6 %) and back pain (3.1 % vs. 2.4 %) the most prevalent [50].

Very recently, Oelke et al. reported the first RCT on tadalafil with an active control group, represented by tamsulosin [51]. A total of 511 men with IPSS higher than 13 and Q_{max} 4 mL/s or higher and 15 mL/s or lower were randomized to a 12-week treatment with tadalafil 5 mg, tamsulosin 0.4, or placebo. The study reconfirmed the improvements in IPSS total score (tadalafil −6.3 vs. tamsulosin −5.7 vs. placebo −4.2), IPSS voiding subscore (tadalafil −4.1 vs. tamsulosin −3.5 vs. placebo −2.6), and IPSS quality-of-life item score (tadalafil −1.3 vs. tamsulosin −1.1 vs. placebo −1.0) over placebo. Notably, the study demonstrated for the first time improvements in Q_{max} (tadalafil 2.4 vs. tamsulosin 2.2 vs. placebo 1.2 mL/s) as compared with placebo, improvements which were similar to those achievable with tamsulosin [51].

The large number of RCTs available on PDE5-Is in male LUTS have been pooled in 2 meta-analyses [44, 52]. Liu et al. demonstrated that PDE5-I were able to improve overall IPSS score of about 2.5 points over placebo (WMD −2.6; 95 % CI, −3.1 to −2.1; $P<0.0001$) in patients with LUTS and with concomitant LUTS and ED [52]. However, meta-analyses reconfirmed the lack of effect on Q_{max} (WMD 0.21; 95 % CI, −0.21 to 0.64; $P=0.32$) and PVR volume (WMD −0.1; 95 % CI, −4.7 to 4.89; $P=0.97$). With regard to AEs, the overall risk of AEs was significantly higher with PDE5-Is than with placebo (37.31 % vs. 24.03 %; relative risk [RR]: 1.87; 95 % CI, 1.31–2.68; $P=0.0005$), although severe AEs were uncommon (sildenafil 1 %, tadalafil 1.1 %, vardenafil 1.8 %) and as prevalent as with placebo (RR: 0.52; 95 % CI, 0.25–1.1; $P=0.07$) [52]. Fairly similar results were provided in another meta-analysis by Gacci et al. [44].

Very limited evidence is currently available on the combination of tadalafil and α-blockers [44]. Among these, 2 small studies reported on the association of alfuzosin and tadalafil [53] and tamsulosin and tadalafil [54], respectively (the combination including other PDE5-Is is not relevant due to the lack of regulatory authority approval for sildenafil and vardenafil in male LUTS). However, the limited number of enrolled patients (20 for each study) does not permit definitive conclusions on the issue.

Thus PDE5-I are effective in improving symptoms in patients with LUTS, with or without concomitant ED. Tadalafil 5 mg is the unique drug in such category to have received FDA and EMEA approvals for such indications and can be used routinely. Although the drug seems not to have an impact on Q_{max}, PVR volume, and other urodynamic parameters as well as the risk of disease progression, it has the significant advantage of improving erectile function in a category of patients at high risk of ED, whereas all the other medical therapies for LUTS can have an impact on sexual function.

Other New Drugs for Male Lower Urinary Tract Symptoms

In the last few years, botulinum toxins have gained popularity for the treatment of neurogenic and nonneurogenic detrusor overactivity and other urologic conditions [55]. A systematic review from Mangera et al. summarized 10 studies evaluating the use of onabotulinumtoxinA and abobotulinumtoxinA in bladder outlet obstruction secondary to BPH, demonstrating significant improvements in total score IPSS (−40 %), Q_{max} (+41 %), PVR volume (−36 %), and quality of life

(+39 %) as well as a reduction in prostate volume (−19 %) and PSA (−13 %) following injection of onabotulinumtoxinA [55]. Unfortunately, only one of these studies was an RCT [56], although of poor methodological quality, which limited the value of the results.

More recently, Marberger et al. reported an elegant phase 2 dose-finding RCT evaluating the efficacy of onabotulinumtoxinA in 380 men 50 years or older with LUTS/BPH, IPSS 12 or higher, total prostate volume 30 to 100 mL, and Q_{max} 5 to 15 mL/s [57]. Specifically, patients were randomized to transrectal or transperineal intraprostatic injection of onabotulinumtoxinA 100 U, 200 U, 300 U, or placebo. The primary efficacy end point was the change from baseline in IPSS at week 12, whereas secondary efficacy end points included IPSS responder analysis (patients with a ≥4-point decrease from baseline in total IPSS), changes from baseline in Q_{max}, prostate volume, transition zone volumes, and PVR volume at week 12.

The study failed to demonstrate any significant impact of onabotulinumtoxinA on IPSS (−6.6 in the 100 U arm vs. −6.3 in the 200 U arm vs. −5.6 in the 300 U arm vs. −5.5 in placebo arm at week 12) as compared with placebo over the 72-week period of evaluation [57]. Although such data sounds discouraging, some other RCTs are still ongoing (e.g., NCT00451191, sponsored by the National Institute of Diabetes and Digestive and Kidney Diseases; NCT01107392, sponsored by Allergan; and NCT01520441), and they will clarify the role of botulinum toxins in LUTS in the near future.

Likely more appealing is the perspective for mirabegron, the first drug of a new class of oral therapy for OAB (i.e., a β3-agonist) to be approved by the US FDA that also received a recommendation for the granting of a marketing authorization from the EMA's Committee for Medicinal Products for Human Use in October 2012. A β3-agonist acts on a totally different molecular pathway. Three subtypes of β-adrenoreceptors (β1, β2, and β3) have been identified in the detrusor muscle and the urothelium, with the β3 subtype the most common in the human detrusor. It has been shown that stimulation of human β3-adrenoreceptors results in direct relaxation of detrusor smooth muscle via activation of G proteins and adenyl cyclase and increases in the levels of cyclic adenosine monophosphate, contributing to urine storage [58].

The results of 2 phase 3 RCTs on mirabegron in OAB syndrome were recently reported [59, 60]. Khullar et al. reported the European and Australian phase 3 registrational study that enrolled more than 2,300 adult patients with micturition frequency of 8 or more times per 24-h period and at least 3 episodes of urgency, with or without incontinence [56]. After placebo run-in, about 2,000 patients were randomized to receive mirabegron 50 mg ($n=497$), mirabegron 100 mg ($n=498$), or tolterodine ER 4 mg ($n=495$) orally once daily for 12 weeks or placebo ($n=497$).

As compared with placebo, patients in both mirabegron arms experienced statistically significant reductions in the mean number of incontinence episodes per 24 h from baseline to final visit (−1.57, −1.46, and −1.17 for mirabegron 50 mg, mirabegron 100 mg, and placebo, respectively; $P<0.05$ for either mirabegron 50 mg or mirabegron 100 mg vs. placebo). Similarly, a statistically significant reduction in the mean number of micturitions per 24 h was observed (−1.93, −1.77, and −1.34

for mirabegron 50 mg, mirabegron 100 mg, and placebo, respectively; $P<0.05$ for either mirabegron 50 mg or mirabegron 100 mg vs. placebo).

Consistent improvements were also found in a broad set of secondary end points. With regard to safety, the incidence of treatment-emergent AEs was similar in all study arms, with mirabegron patients failing to experience more cardiovascular AEs than placebo (as well as all the typical AEs of anticholinergics) [56].

In the second phase 3 RCT, Chapple et al. evaluated long-term safety and efficacy of mirabegron [60]. More than 2,400 patients were randomized to receive mirabegron 50 mg ($n=812$), mirabegron 100 mg ($n=812$), or tolterodine ER 4 mg ($n=812$) orally once daily for 12 months, with the primary end point to evaluate the incidence and severity of AEs. Notably, about 81 % of the patients included in the study were not treatment naive but had previously been included in the 2 US and European-Australian registrational phase 3 RCTs. The prevalence of AEs was about 60 % in each study arm, with most mild to moderate, and discontinuation rates were about 6 % in each arm over the 12-month treatment [60].

Taken together, the data of the available studies suggest that mirabegron is the first drug that will soon be available on the market of a new category of oral drugs for OAB syndrome with good efficacy in improving symptoms (at least until the tested 12-month time frame) and a favorable placebo-like profile of AEs. Considering the increasing interest in bladder function in LUTS patients, as well as the high prevalence of patients with storage symptoms and the relative efficacy of anticholinergic drugs, it is easy to hypothesize that mirabegron and eventually other β3 agonists will be soon tested in male LUTS suggestive of BPH.

Other possible drugs for BPH are luteinizing hormone-releasing hormone (LHRH) antagonists. Similar to prostate cancer, the rationale for their use is based on inhibiting LHRH receptors in the pituitary, thereby blocking the signal for testosterone production in the testes and consequently inhibiting prostate growth. Clinical studies have shown that cetrorelix decreases prostate volume and improves LUTS in patients experiencing BPH. However, the efficacy of LHRH antagonists in symptom relief is only mild, and the antiandrogenic side effects such as impotence are typically considered unacceptable for BPH therapy [61].

Several other molecular pathways are objects of intense clinical research aimed at identifying new drugs for BPH. P2X1-purinoceptor antagonists, adenosine receptor antagonists, cannabinoids, α-adrenoceptor-interacting proteins, RhoA/Rho kinase, vitamin D3 analogs, progestogens, carotenoids, pomegranate, and many more molecules have been actively investigated [61, 62], but none of these drugs have reached the level of phase 3 RCTs.

NX-1207 is an apoptosis-inducing agent developed by Nymox Pharmaceutical Corporation that has been tested in both phase 2 and phase 3 studies. Injected intraprostatically, NX-1207 was shown to reduce prostate volume in animal studies. In phase 2 studies, the 2.5-mg dose was shown to be significantly more effective than placebo in improving AUA-SI (-11.0 points; P vs. placebo 0.008). In another phase 2 study, 2.5 mg NX-1207 injection was compared with short-term therapy with finasteride, resulting in being noninferior [63]. Based on those promising data, several North American phase 3 trials are underway (NCT00918983, NCT00945490) in patients with LUTS/BPH to assess safety, as well as effect on symptoms, prostate volume, and urinary Q_{max} [62].

Conclusions

Medical treatment of male LUTS suggestive of BPH can be based on several effective drugs able to improve patient symptoms, reduce the risk of complications, and reduce the incidence of BPH-related surgery. On the whole, such drugs are quite well tolerated, although ED and ejaculatory dysfunction may be a significant concern, in both young patients who are more frequently sexually active or in elderly patients with concomitant ED. However, it must be kept in mind that the extent of symptom relief achievable with any drug therapy is significantly lower than those achievable with standard prostatic surgery.

References

1. Oelke M, Bachmann A, Descazeaud M, Emberton S, Gravas MC, Michel J, N'Dow J, Nordling JJ de la Rosette. Guidelines on the management of male lower urinary tract symptoms (LUTS), incl. benign prostatic obstruction (BPO). Available from: http://www.uroweb.org/gls/pdf/12_Male_LUTS_after.corrections.pdf.
2. McVary KT, Roehrborn CG, Avins AL, Barry MJ, Bruskewitz RC, Donnell RF, et al. Update on AUA guideline on the management of benign prostatic hyperplasia. J Urol. 2011;185(5):1793–803.
3. National Institute for Health and Clinical Excellence guidelines. The management of lower urinary tract symptoms in men. Available from: http://guidance.nice.org.uk/CG97/NICEGuidance/pdf/English.
4. Brown CT, Yap T, Cromwell DA, Rixon L, Steed L, Mulligan K, et al. Self management for men with lower urinary tract symptoms: randomised controlled trial. BMJ. 2007;334(7583):25. PubMed PMID: 17118949. Pubmed Central PMCID: 1764065.
5. Cornu JN, Cussenot O, Haab F, Lukacs B. A widespread population study of actual medical management of lower urinary tract symptoms related to benign prostatic hyperplasia across Europe and beyond official clinical guidelines. Eur Urol. 2010;58(3):450–6. PubMed PMID: 20554374.
6. Schilit S, Benzeroual KE. Silodosin: a selective alpha1A-adrenergic receptor antagonist for the treatment of benign prostatic hyperplasia. Clin Ther. 2009;31(11):2489–502. PubMed PMID: 20109995. Epub 2010/01/30. eng.
7. Wilt TJ, Howe RW, Rutks IR, MacDonald R. Terazosin for benign prostatic hyperplasia. Cochrane Database Syst Rev (Online). 2002;(4):CD003851. PubMed PMID: 12519611. Epub 2003/01/10. eng.
8. Wilt TJ, Mac Donald R, Rutks I. Tamsulosin for benign prostatic hyperplasia. Cochrane Database Syst Rev (Online). 2003;(1):CD002081. PubMed PMID: 12535426. Epub 2003/01/22. eng.
9. Marks LS, Gittelman MC, Hill LA, Volinn W, Hoel G. Rapid efficacy of the highly selective alpha1A-adrenoceptor antagonist silodosin in men with signs and symptoms of benign prostatic hyperplasia: pooled results of 2 phase 3 studies. J Urol. 2009;181(6):2634–40. PubMed PMID: 19371887. Epub 2009/04/18. eng.

10. Kawabe K, Yoshida M, Homma Y, Silodosin Clinical Study G. Silodosin, a new alpha1A-adrenoceptor-selective antagonist for treating benign prostatic hyperplasia: results of a phase III randomized, placebo-controlled, double-blind study in Japanese men. BJU Int. 2006;98(5):1019–24.
11. Chapple CR, Montorsi F, Tammela TL, Wirth M, Koldewijn E, Fernandez Fernandez E, et al. Silodosin therapy for lower urinary tract symptoms in men with suspected benign prostatic hyperplasia: results of an international, randomized, double-blind, placebo- and active-controlled clinical trial performed in Europe. Eur Urol. 2011;59(3):342–52. PubMed PMID: 21109344.
12. Novara G, Tubaro A, Sanseverino R, Spatafora S, Artibani W, Zattoni F, et al. Systematic review and meta-analysis of randomized controlled trials evaluating silodosin in the treatment of non-neurogenic male lower urinary tract symptoms suggestive of benign prostatic enlargement. World J Urol. 2013;31(4):997–1008. PubMed PMID: 23053207. Epub 2012/10/12. Eng.
13. Gormley GJ, Stoner E, Bruskewitz RC, Imperato-McGinley J, Walsh PC, McConnell JD, et al. The effect of finasteride in men with benign prostatic hyperplasia. The Finasteride Study Group. N Engl J Med. 1992;327(17):1185–91. PubMed PMID: 1383816. Epub 1992/10/22. eng.
14. Tenover JL, Pagano GA, Morton AS, Liss CL, Byrnes CA. Efficacy and tolerability of finasteride in symptomatic benign prostatic hyperplasia: a primary care study. Primary Care Investigator Study Group. Clin Ther. 1997;19(2):243–58. PubMed PMID: 9152564. Epub 1997/03/01. eng.
15. Finasteride (MK-906) in the treatment of benign prostatic hyperplasia. The Finasteride Study Group. Prostate. 1993;22(4):291–9. PubMed PMID: 7684524. Epub 1993/01/01. eng.
16. Byrnes CA, Morton AS, Liss CL, Lippert MC, Gillenwater JY. Efficacy, tolerability, and effect on health-related quality of life of finasteride versus placebo in men with symptomatic benign prostatic hyperplasia: a community based study. CUSP Investigators. Community based study of Proscar. Clin Ther. 1995;17(5):956–69. PubMed PMID: 8595647. Epub 1995/09/01. eng.
17. McConnell JD, Bruskewitz R, Walsh P, Andriole G, Lieber M, Holtgrewe HL, et al. The effect of finasteride on the risk of acute urinary retention and the need for surgical treatment among men with benign prostatic hyperplasia. Finasteride Long-Term Efficacy and Safety Study Group. N Engl J Med. 1998;338(9):557–63. PubMed PMID: 9475762. Epub 1998/02/26. eng.
18. Roehrborn CG, Boyle P, Nickel JC, Hoefner K, Andriole G, Aria A, et al. Efficacy and safety of a dual inhibitor of 5-alpha-reductase types 1 and 2 (dutasteride) in men with benign prostatic hyperplasia. Urology. 2002;60(3):434–41. PubMed PMID: 12350480.
19. Tacklind J, Fink HA, Macdonald R, Rutks I, Wilt TJ. Finasteride for benign prostatic hyperplasia. Cochrane Database Syst Rev (Online). 2010 (10):CD006015. PubMed PMID: 20927745. Epub 2010/10/12. eng.
20. Lepor H, Williford WO, Barry MJ, Brawer MK, Dixon CM, Gormley G, et al. The efficacy of terazosin, finasteride, or both in benign prostatic hyperplasia. Veterans Affairs Cooperative Studies Benign Prostatic Hyperplasia Study Group. N Engl J Med. 1996;335(8):533–9. PubMed PMID: 8684407. Epub 1996/08/22. eng.
21. Debruyne FM, Jardin A, Colloi D, Resel L, Witjes WP, Delauche-Cavallier MC, et al. Sustained-release alfuzosin, finasteride and the combination of both in the treatment of benign prostatic hyperplasia. European ALFIN Study Group. Eur Urol. 1998;34(3):169–75. PubMed PMID: 9732187. Epub 1998/09/10. eng.
22. Kirby RS, Roehrborn C, Boyle P, Bartsch G, Jardin A, Cary MM, et al. Efficacy and tolerability of doxazosin and finasteride, alone or in combination, in treatment of symptomatic benign prostatic hyperplasia: the Prospective European Doxazosin and Combination Therapy (PREDICT) trial. Urology. 2003;61(1):119–26. PubMed PMID: 12559281. Epub 2003/02/01. eng.
23. McConnell JD, Roehrborn CG, Bautista OM, Andriole Jr GL, Dixon CM, Kusek JW, et al. The long-term effect of doxazosin, finasteride, and combination therapy on the clinical progression of benign prostatic hyperplasia. N Engl J Med. 2003;349(25):2387–98. PubMed PMID: 14681504.

24. Crawford ED, Wilson SS, McConnell JD, Slawin KM, Lieber MC, Smith JA, et al. Baseline factors as predictors of clinical progression of benign prostatic hyperplasia in men treated with placebo. J Urol. 2006;175(4):1422–6; discussion 6–7. PubMed PMID: 16516013.
25. Kaplan SA, McConnell JD, Roehrborn CG, Meehan AG, Lee MW, Noble WR, et al. Combination therapy with doxazosin and finasteride for benign prostatic hyperplasia in patients with lower urinary tract symptoms and a baseline total prostate volume of 25 ml or greater. J Urol. 2006;175(1):217–20; discussion 20–1. PubMed PMID: 16406915.
26. Roehrborn CG, Siami P, Barkin J, Damiao R, Major-Walker K, Nandy I, et al. The effects of combination therapy with dutasteride and tamsulosin on clinical outcomes in men with symptomatic benign prostatic hyperplasia: 4-year results from the CombAT study. Eur Urol. 2010;57(1):123–31. PubMed PMID: 19825505.
27. Novara G, Galfano A, Secco S, D'Elia C, Cavalleri S, Ficarra V, et al. A systematic review and meta-analysis of randomized controlled trials with antimuscarinic drugs for overactive bladder. Eur Urol. 2008;54(4):740–63. PubMed PMID: 18632201. Epub 2008/07/18. eng.
28. Kaplan SA, Roehrborn CG, Rovner ES, Carlsson M, Bavendam T, Guan Z. Tolterodine and tamsulosin for treatment of men with lower urinary tract symptoms and overactive bladder: a randomized controlled trial. JAMA. 2006;296(19):2319–28. PubMed PMID: 17105794. Epub 2006/11/16. eng.
29. Van Kerrebroeck P, Haab F, Angulo JC, Vik V, Katona F, Garcia-Hernandez A, Klaver M, Traudtner K, Oelke M. Efficacy and safety of solifenacin pl 1 us tamsulosin OCAS™ in men with LUTS associated with BPH: results from a phase 2, dose-finding study (SATURN). Eur Urol. 2013;64(3):398–407.
30. Chapple C, Herschorn S, Abrams P, Sun F, Brodsky M, Guan Z. Tolterodine treatment improves storage symptoms suggestive of overactive bladder in men treated with alpha-blockers. Eur Urol. 2009;56(3):534–41. PubMed PMID: 19070418. Epub 2008/12/17. eng.
31. Kaplan SA, McCammon K, Fincher R, Fakhoury A, He W. Safety and tolerability of solifenacin add-on therapy to alpha-blocker treated men with residual urgency and frequency. J Urol. 2013;189(1 Suppl):S129–34. PubMed PMID: 23234618. Epub 2012/12/19. eng.
32. Geavlete P, Multescu R, Geavlete B. Serenoa repens extract in the treatment of benign prostatic hyperplasia. Ther Adv Urol. 2011;3(4):193–8. PubMed PMID: 21969849. Pubmed Central PMCID: PMC3175703. Epub 2011/10/05. eng.
33. Tacklind J, MacDonald R, Rutks I, Wilt TJ. Serenoa repens for benign prostatic hyperplasia. Cochrane Database Syst Rev (Online). 2009; (2):CD001423. PubMed PMID: 19370565. Pubmed Central PMCID: PMC3090655. Epub 2009/04/17. eng.
34. Barry MJ, Meleth S, Lee JY, Kreder KJ, Avins AL, Nickel JC, et al. Effect of increasing doses of saw palmetto extract on lower urinary tract symptoms: a randomized trial. JAMA. 2011;306(12):1344–51. PubMed PMID: 21954478. Pubmed Central PMCID: 3326341.
35. Habib FK, Wyllie MG. Not all brands are created equal: a comparison of selected components of different brands of Serenoa repens extract. Prostate Cancer Prostatic Dis. 2004;7(3):195–200.
36. Scaglione F, Lucini V, Pannacci M, Caronno A, Leone C. Comparison of the potency of different brands of Serenoa repens extract on 5alpha-reductase types I and II in prostatic co-cultured epithelial and fibroblast cells. Pharmacology. 2008;82(4):270–5.
37. Glemain P, Coulange C, Billebaud T, Gattegno B, Muszynski R, Loeb G. Tamsulosin with or without Serenoa repens in benign prostatic hyperplasia: the OCOS trial. Prog Urol. 2002;12(3):395–403; discussion 4. PubMed PMID: 12189745. Epub 2002/08/23. Tamsulosine avec ou sans Serenoa repens dans l'hypertrophie benigne de la prostate: l'essai OCOS. fre.
38. Hizli F, Uygur MC. A prospective study of the efficacy of Serenoa repens, Tamsulosin, and Serenoa repens plus Tamsulosin treatment for patients with benign prostate hyperplasia. Int Urol Nephrol. 2007;39(3):879–86.
39. Rosen R, Altwein J, Boyle P, Kirby RS, Lukacs B, Meuleman E, et al. Lower urinary tract symptoms and male sexual dysfunction: the multinational survey of the aging male (MSAM-7). Eur Urol. 2003;44(6):637–49. PubMed PMID: 14644114.
40. Andersson KE, de Groat WC, McVary KT, Lue TF, Maggi M, Roehrborn CG, et al. Tadalafil for the treatment of lower urinary tract symptoms secondary to benign prostatic hyperplasia:

pathophysiology and mechanism(s) of action. Neurouroluro dynamics. 2011;30(3):292–301. PubMed PMID: 21284024. Epub 2011/02/02. eng.
41. McVary KT, Kaufman J, Young JM, Tseng LJ. Sildenafil citrate improves erectile function: a randomised double-blind trial with open-label extension. Int J Clin Pract. 2007;61(11): 1843–9. PubMed PMID: 17887993. Epub 2007/09/25. eng.
42. Sairam K, Kulinskaya E, McNicholas TA, Boustead GB, Hanbury DC. Sildenafil influences lower urinary tract symptoms. BJU Int. 2002;90(9):836–9. PubMed PMID: 12460342. Epub 2002/12/04. eng.
43. Martinez-Salamanca JI, Carballido J, Eardley I, Giuliano F, Gratzke C, Rosen R, et al. Phosphodiesterase type 5 inhibitors in the management of non-neurogenic male lower urinary tract symptoms: critical analysis of current evidence. Eur Urol. 2011;60(3):527–35. PubMed PMID: 21684677. Epub 2011/06/21. eng.
44. Gacci M, Corona G, Salvi M, Vignozzi L, McVary KT, Kaplan SA, et al. A systematic review and meta-analysis on the use of phosphodiesterase 5 inhibitors alone or in combination with alpha-blockers for lower urinary tract symptoms due to benign prostatic hyperplasia. Eur Urol. 2012;61(5):994–1003. PubMed PMID: 22405510. Epub 2012/03/13. eng.
45. Stief CG, Porst H, Neuser D, Beneke M, Ulbrich E. A randomised, placebo-controlled study to assess the efficacy of twice-daily vardenafil in the treatment of lower urinary tract symptoms secondary to benign prostatic hyperplasia. Eur Urol. 2008;53(6):1236–44. PubMed PMID: 18281145. Epub 2008/02/19. eng.
46. Hatzimouratidis K, Hatzichristou DG. Looking to the future for erectile dysfunction therapies. Drugs. 2008;68(2):231–50. PubMed PMID: 18197727.
47. Wrishko R, Sorsaburu S, Wong D, Strawbridge A, McGill J. Safety, efficacy, and pharmacokinetic overview of low-dose daily administration of tadalafil. J Sex Med. 2009;6(7):2039–48. PubMed PMID: 19453893. Epub 2009/05/21. eng.
48. McVary KT, Roehrborn CG, Kaminetsky JC, Auerbach SM, Wachs B, Young JM, et al. Tadalafil relieves lower urinary tract symptoms secondary to benign prostatic hyperplasia. J Urol. 2007;177(4):1401–7. PubMed PMID: 17382741. Epub 2007/03/27. eng.
49. Roehrborn CG, McVary KT, Elion-Mboussa A, Viktrup L. Tadalafil administered once daily for lower urinary tract symptoms secondary to benign prostatic hyperplasia: a dose finding study. J Urology. 2008;180(4):1228–34. PubMed PMID: 18722631. Epub 2008/08/30. eng.
50. Porst H, Kim ED, Casabe AR, Mirone V, Secrest RJ, Xu L, et al. Efficacy and safety of tadalafil once daily in the treatment of men with lower urinary tract symptoms suggestive of benign prostatic hyperplasia: results of an international randomized, double-blind, placebo-controlled trial. Eur Urol. 2011;60(5):1105–13. PubMed PMID: 21871706. Epub 2011/08/30. eng.
51. Oelke M, Giuliano F, Mirone V, Xu L, Cox D, Viktrup L. Monotherapy with tadalafil or tamsulosin similarly improved lower urinary tract symptoms suggestive of benign prostatic hyperplasia in an international, randomised, parallel, placebo-controlled clinical trial. Eur Urol. 2012;61(5):917–25. PubMed PMID: 22297243. Epub 2012/02/03. eng.
52. Liu L, Zheng S, Han P, Wei Q. Phosphodiesterase-5 inhibitors for lower urinary tract symptoms secondary to benign prostatic hyperplasia: a systematic review and meta-analysis. Urology. 2011;77(1):123–9. PubMed PMID: 21195830.
53. Liguori G, Trombetta C, De Giorgi G, Pomara G, Maio G, Vecchio D, et al. Efficacy and safety of combined oral therapy with tadalafil and alfuzosin: an integrated approach to the management of patients with lower urinary tract symptoms and erectile dysfunction. J Sex Med. 2009;6(2):544–52. PubMed PMID: 19138360. Epub 2009/01/14. eng.
54. Bechara A, Romano S, Casabe A, Haime S, Dedola P, Hernandez C, et al. Comparative efficacy assessment of tamsulosin vs. tamsulosin plus tadalafil in the treatment of LUTS/BPH. Pilot study. J Sex Med. 2008;5(9):2170–8. PubMed PMID: 18638006. Epub 2008/07/22. eng.
55. Mangera A, Andersson KE, Apostolidis A, Chapple C, Dasgupta P, Giannantoni A, et al. Contemporary management of lower urinary tract disease with botulinum toxin A: a systematic review of botox (onabotulinumtoxinA) and dysport (abobotulinumtoxinA). Eur Urol. 2011;60(4):784–95. PubMed PMID: 21782318.

56. Maria G, Brisinda G, Civello IM, Bentivoglio AR, Sganga G, Albanese A. Relief by botulinum toxin of voiding dysfunction due to benign prostatic hyperplasia: results of a randomized, placebo-controlled study. Urology. 2003;62(2):259–64; discussion 64–5. PubMed PMID: 12893330.
57. Marberger M, Chartier-Kastler E, Egerdie B, Lee KS, Grosse J, Bugarin D, et al. A randomized double-blind placebo-controlled phase 2 dose-ranging study of OnabotulinumtoxinA in men with benign prostatic hyperplasia. Eur Urol. 2013;63(3):496–503. PubMed PMID: 23098762.
58. Aizawa N, Homma Y, Igawa Y. Effects of mirabegron, a novel beta3-adrenoceptor agonist, on primary bladder afferent activity and bladder microcontractions in rats compared with the effects of oxybutynin. Eur Urol. 2012;62(6):1165–73. PubMed PMID: 22981677. Epub 2012/09/18. eng.
59. Khullar V, Amarenco G, Angulo JC, Cambronero J, Hoye K, Milsom I, et al. Efficacy and tolerability of mirabegron, a beta(3)-adrenoceptor agonist, in patients with overactive bladder: results from a randomised European-Australian phase 3 trial. Eur Urol. 2013;63(2):283–95. PubMed PMID: 23182126.
60. Chapple CR, Kaplan SA, Mitcheson D, Klecka J, Cummings J, Drogendijk T, et al. Randomized double-blind, active-controlled phase 3 study to assess 12-month safety and efficacy of mirabegron, a beta(3)-adrenoceptor agonist, in overactive bladder. Eur Urol. 2013;63(2):296–305. PubMed PMID: 23195283.
61. Ventura S, Oliver VL, White CW, Xie JH, Haynes JM, Exintaris B. Novel drug targets for the pharmacotherapy of benign prostatic hyperplasia (BPH). Br J Pharmacol. 2011;163(5):891–907.
62. Hashim H, Abrams P. Emerging drugs for the treatment of benign prostatic obstruction. Expert Opin Emerg Drugs. 2010;15(2):159–74.
63. Shore N. NX-1207: a novel investigational drug for the treatment of benign prostatic hyperplasia. Expert Opin Investig Drugs. 2010;19(2):305–10.

Chapter 6
Open Prostatectomy and Standard Endosurgery

Riccardo Autorino and Cosimo De Nunzio

Abstract Given the widespread use of medical therapies and the introduction of a myriad of minimally invasive treatments, the patient population undergoing the most established surgical procedures for BPO has considerably changed over the last two decades. General indications for surgical intervention are well described in current guidelines. However, patients may seek surgery as primary treatment, and the decision for surgery should be always based on the patient's risk/benefit assessment. TURP is still considered as the gold standard treatment, given its well-documented long-term efficacy. Moreover, its surgical-related morbidity has been considerably reduced with introduction of bipolar systems. Simple prostatectomy can have a role in certain instances as it also appears to be safe and effective in contemporary series, especially in settings where more recent (laser) technology is not available. TUIP can be regarded as a viable option in selected patient with a suitable gland. Other recently introduced electrosurgical options, such as TUERP and TURisV, seem promising and user-friendly, but they need to be further scrutinized.

Keywords Benign prostatic obstruction • Surgical treatment • Simple prostatectomy • Transurethral resection of the prostate • Transurethral incision of the prostate

---

R. Autorino (✉)
Urology Unit, Second University of Naples, Naples, Italy

YAU-EAU BPH group, Italy
e-mail: ricautor@gmail.com

C. De Nunzio
Department of Urology, Ospedale Sant'Andrea,
University "La Sapienza", Rome, Italy

YAU-EAU BPH group, Italy
e-mail: cosimodenunzio@virgilio.it

Table 6.1 Current recommendations for surgery in patients with BPO

	Recommendation
EAU [4]	Surgical management is an appropriate treatment for men with moderate/severe LUTS who (i) did not improve after medical therapy, (ii) do not want medical therapy yet request active intervention, and (iii) present with a strong indication for surgery (refractory urinary retention, renal insufficiency, bladder stones, recurrent urinary tract infection, recurrent hematuria refractory to medical treatment with 5ARIs)
AUA [6]	Surgery is recommended for patients who have renal insufficiency secondary to BPH, who have recurrent urinary tract infections (UTIs), gross hematuria due to BPH, or bladder stones, and who have LUTS refractory to other therapies. The presence of a bladder diverticulum is not an absolute indication for surgery unless associated with recurrent UTI or progressive bladder dysfunction
JUA [5]	Surgical treatment for BPH is indicated in cases of (i) insufficient response to medical therapy, (ii) the presence of moderate to severe symptoms, and (iii) in the presence of (or concern about) comorbidities, such as urinary retention, UTI, hematuria, and bladder stones

EAU European Association of Urology, *AUA* American Urological Association, *JUA* Japanese Urological Association

Introduction

Significant changes in the management of symptomatic benign prostatic enlargement (BPE) and obstruction (BPO) have occurred over the past 20 years. Most patients are nowadays started on pharmacological therapy, and this conservative approach has resulted in patients presenting for surgery at an older age with more comorbidities and larger prostates than usual after an unsuccessful pharmacological therapy [1]. Thus, failure of medical therapy has now become one of the most important indications for surgical treatment, and those undergoing the procedure experience more progression events (e.g., acute or chronic urinary retention), poorer immediate short-term results, and higher rates of postoperative complications than those who had the operation two decades previously [2]. Although alpha1-blockers delayed the need for surgery by a few years, patients with a large prostate volume might ultimately need to undergo surgery [3].

Open prostatectomy represents the oldest surgical treatment modality for lower urinary tract symptoms (LUTS) secondary to benign prostatic obstruction (BPO). Transurethral resection of the prostate (TURP) still represents the reference standard among the surgical options. General indications for surgical intervention are well described in current guidelines (Table 6.1) [4–6]. However, patients may seek surgery as primary treatment, and the decision for surgery should be always based on the patient's risk/benefit assessment.

Open (Simple) Prostatectomy

Different techniques have been described to perform open (simple) prostatectomy. The suprapubic (transvesical) approach for open prostatectomy was initially used by Fuller in the USA [7] and McGill in the UK [8], but the results were poor. Sir

Peter Freyer described his method of suprapubic prostatectomy (the so-called Freyer's transvesical prostatectomy) in four cases, published in the *British Medical Journal* in 1901 [9], and he updated his series in 1912 when he published the outcomes from his first 1,000 operations [10]. The technique includes a transverse incision made in the anterior bladder wall, then the index finger is then placed in the urethra, and with forward pressure towards the symphysis, the urethral mucosa is broken, and the plane between the surgical capsule and the adenomas is defined, then the prostatic adenomas are then bluntly separated from the capsule with the finger. Hemostatic sutures are placed in the posterior corners of the cavity and the posterior margin, taking care not to include the ureteral orifices. Postoperative hemostasis might be obtained using gauze packing and/or traction on a large balloon catheter.

In 1945, Terence Millin reported in *The Lancet* a novel retropubic approach for enucleation of the prostate in 20 nonselected consecutive cases [11]. The *Millin prostatectomy* revolutionized surgery for BPH, but also the surgical treatment of prostate cancer, as Millin's retropubic approach became rapidly popular [12]. In this procedure, a transverse incision is made in the anterior prostatic capsule, and the adenomas freed bluntly with a scissor and the index finger. The prostatic capsule is closed after insertion of a transurethral balloon catheter for drainage.

A third approach to the removal of the enlarged prostate was via the perineum – the so-called *perineal* prostatectomy, which was introduced by Hugh Young in Baltimore (USA), in 1903 [13], but it never become popular compared to the other routes.

Despite being regarded as a procedure that can completely relieve BPO, open prostatectomy is nowadays used less frequently. Bruskewitz et al. reported that open prostatectomy comprises 3 % of the prostatectomies performed in the USA [14]. Lukacs [15] and Ahlstrand et al. [16] reported that 14 and 12 % of BPH surgical procedures in France and Sweden, respectively, were open prostatectomy. However, open prostatectomy was reported to be used at considerable higher rates in other studies. Serretta et al. demonstrated a 32 % rate of in a study from southern Italy [17], and open prostatectomy rate reached 40 % in Israel [18]. In a more recent survey conducted in Japan to investigate the trend in surgical procedures for BPH during the past 10 years, Masumori et al. found that open prostatectomy was still a viable option in 2009, with 555 procedures out of 20,413 (2,7 %) [19]. When considering patients with prostate volume over 100 mL, open prostatectomy was indicated by 46 % of the surveyed urology centers.

Traditionally, indications mainly consist of large adenoma (>80–100 cc), especially when there is a coexistent pathology that is easily managed transvesically, such as large bladder diverticulum or multiple bladder stones [20]. It can be also considered in patients with unilateral or bilateral inguinal hernias, as these can be repaired preperitoneally at the same time through the same incision. Another indication for open prostatectomy is ankylosis of the hips, preventing proper placement of the patient in the dorsal lithotomy position for TURP. The choice of whether to perform the operation in a retropubic or suprapubic (transvesical) manner remains controversial and depends on surgeon training or comfort. The suprapubic approach is preferred by most if there is an extremely large median lobe, concomitant bladder stones, or a bladder diverticulum requiring repair. The advantages of the retropubic technique include improved anatomic prostatic exposure, direct visualization of the adenoma during enucleation to ensure complete removal and direct visualization of the prostate fossa after enucleation for hemorrhage control, precise division of the prostatic urethra optimizing preservation of urinary continence, and minimal or no surgical trauma to the bladder. The benefits of the perineal approach are the ability to avoid the retropubic space which can be useful when there is a history of prior retropubic surgery; the ability to treat clinically significant prostatic abscess and cysts; and less postoperative pain; more suitable in obese patients [21].

There is a paucity of contemporary Western literature pertaining to open simple prostatectomy. Most references refer to old Western series or contemporary experience from developing nations lacking access to modern TURP technology. There are also few data in the recent literature about the long-term efficacy of open prostatectomy. Nevertheless, available evidence proves that open prostatectomy is mainly performed through the suprapubic technique and it represents an effective procedure with a low rate of complications and a durable success (Table 6.2) [17, 22–29].

The Calabro-Sicilian Society of Urology published one of the major present day series of simple prostatectomies performed between 1997 and 1998 [17]. Open prostatectomy accounted for 32 % ($n=1,804$) of all surgical treatment during the study period. The postoperative median hospitalization time was 7 days. Concomitant lower urinary tract disease was present in 25 % of the patients. Severe bleeding occurred in 11.6 % of open prostatectomies. Blood transfusions were given in 8.2 % of cases. Sepsis was reported in 8.6 % of the patients. Re-interventions, within 2 years, mainly due to bladder neck stenosis, were reported in 3.6 % of cases.

In a landmark study, Madersbacher et al. reported a nationwide analysis on over 20,000 cases looking at the long-term rates of reoperation, myocardial infarction, and mortality after TURP and open prostatectomy [30]. Actuarial cumulative incidences of a secondary TURP after primary TURP at 1, 5, and 8 years were 2.9, 5.8, and 7.4 %; the respective numbers after open prostatectomy are 1.0, 2.7, and 3.4 %. This study showed a higher reoperation rate after TURP compared to open prostatectomy.

Perioperative hemorrhage represents a major problem of open prostatectomy. Thus, different methods have been proposed to optimize the control of bleeding. Modifications of the classical Millin retropubic were described by Gregoir [31], who recommended a preventive ligation of the prostatic arterial pedicles; by Walsh and Oesterling [32], who incised the puboprostatic ligaments and used a mass-clamp ligature of the deep dorsal vein complex at a more distal level and also recommended wider ligature of the lateral prostatic pedicles at the vesicoprostatic junction; and by Amen-Palma and Arteaga [33], who described a modification in which the lateral pedicles and vessels of the penile dorsal vein complex were sutured only after enucleating the adenoma. A more recent modification was proposed by Srougi et al. [34]. These authors used a wide ligature at the posterolateral aspect of the vesicoprostatic junction, additional ligatures applied on each side at a more posterior position, and a series of hemostatic sutures applied in the anterior prostatic surface. They reported a prospective randomized analysis of 62 men with BPH who

6 Open Prostatectomy and Standard Endosurgery

Table 6.2 Open simple prostatectomy: literature overview

Reference	No. of pts	Age, years	Technique	Surgical outcomes EPW/S	CR, %	TR, %	MR, %	CT, days	HS, days	Functional parameters after surgery SS	PVR, ml	Qmax, ml/s
Meier et al. [22]	240	nr	SP	61 g	19.6	4.6	0	7	nr	nr	nr	nr
Condie et al. [23]	200	64	SP	nr	14	1	1	7	6.2	nr	nr	nr
Tubaro et al. [24]	32	69.5	SP	63 g	31.3	0	0	5.4	6.2	1.5[a]	8	29
Serretta et al. [17]	1,804	68.5	SP and RP	75 ml	nr	8.2	0.05	5.5	6.9	nr	nr	nr
Varkarakis et al. [25]	232	72.6	SP	104 ml	20.6	6.8	0	5	6	1.7[a]	11.9	23.7
Adam et al. [60]	201	70	SP	63.5 g	nr	18.9	0	6	10	4^	0[b]	20.8[b]
Helfand et al. [27]	56	70.9	SP and RP	112 ml	32.1	7.1	0	4.7	6.7	4^	5.3	nr
Gratzke et al. [28]	902	71.3	nr	84.8 g	17.3	7.5	0.2	nr	11.9	17.5	23.1
Suer et al. [29]	664	67.5	SP and RP	88.7 g	18.5	12.7	0.3	8	6.7	10.6	28	23.7

Values expressed as means (standard deviation) unless otherwise specified
nr not reported, *SP* suprapubic, *RP* retropubic, *EPW* estimated prostate weight (size), *CR* complication rate, *TR* transfusion rate (allogenic), *MR* mortality rate, *CT* catheterization time, *HS* hospital stay, *SS* Symptom Score, *PVR* post-void residual urine, Q_{max} maximum flow rate
[a]IPSS; ^AUA-SI
[b]Median values

Table 6.3 Open prostatectomy versus TURP: available level 1 evidence

	Simforoosh et al. [39]		Ou et al. [40]	
	OP	TURP	OP	TURP
No. of pts	50	49	34	35
Age, years	71.7	61	71.3	70.9
Prostate size, cc	47.9	44.4	138.4	131
Prostate weight, g	34.5	31	116.8	69.7
Catheter time, days	7	5	7.5	4.1
HS, days	nr	nr	9.2	5.6
Follow-up, months	12		12	
IPSS improvement, %	82.3	75.2	87.6	62.3
PFR improvement, %	157	100	230	102
PVR improvement, %	96.7	100	88.6	70.5
Transfusion rate, %	8	10	11.7	14.2
Mortality rate, %	2	0	0	0
Reoperation rate, %	0	16	0	5.7

Values expressed as mean (standard deviation) unless otherwise specified

nr not reported, *OP* open transvesical prostatectomy, *TURP* transurethral resection of the prostate, *IPSS* International Prostate Symptom Score, *PFR* peak flow rate, *PVR* post-void residual urine

consecutively had simple prostatectomy and were randomized to a Millin modified retropubic prostatectomy or a classical transvesical prostatectomy [35]. The median blood loss during surgery was lower with the modified Millin technique (median 362 vs 640 mL, $p = 0.007$), as well as the transfusion rates, when compared to the classic transvesical prostatectomy. Shaheen and Quinlan also advocated an early vascular control, by ligating the dorsal venous plexus, bilaterally clamping the internal iliac arteries, and ligating the inferior vesical vessels, in order to minimize the blood loss during either Millin or Freyer prostatectomy [36].

With the aim of avoiding urethral catheter-related complications, Djaladat et al. successfully performed a catheter-free suprapubic prostatectomy by using a special handmade cystostomy catheter [37]. More recently, Okorie et al. determine whether postoperative bladder irrigation following suprapubic prostatectomy can be safely eliminated by modifying the bladder neck repair technique [38].

RCTs comparing open prostatectomy versus TURP remain scanty (Table 6.3). Simforoosh et al. compared the two procedures for prostates sized 30–70 g by enrolling 100 patients [39]. Improvement of peak flow rate was higher for open prostatectomy (median 11.1 vs. 8.0 ml/s; $p = .02$). Reoperation due to residual prostate lobe, urethral stricture, and urinary retention was performed in eight patients in TURP group (16 %) versus none in prostatectomy group ($p = 0.006$). Hospitalization duration was slightly longer in patients undergoing open surgery ($p = 0.04$). Ou et al. compared in a prospective randomized trial the safety and efficacy of transvesical prostatectomy and TURP in a different population, i.e., for prostate greater than 80 mL [40]. Of 80 patients eligible to participate, 69 patients completed 12 months of follow-up. More prostatic tissue was resected during the open procedure (84.4 %

vs. 53.2 %; $p<0.001$). IPSS, Q_{max}, and PVR volume were significantly better in the open prostatectomy group. Two TURP patients developed urethral stricture requiring reoperation. Thus, the authors concluded that the open procedure seems to be more effective and safer than TURP when prostate volume is >80 mL.

EAU guidelines, as well as those from other major urological associations, still recognize a role for open prostatectomy in the management of BPH patients [4–6, 41, 42] (Table 6.4).

TURP

Since its first description in 1932 [43], the basic principle of TURP has remained unchanged, which is the removal of tissue from the transition zone of the prostate to reduce BPO and, consequently, to reduce LUTS.

During the last decade, there has been a continuous decline in the rate of TURPs performed. In 1999, TURP represented 81 % of all surgery for BPH in the USA, but, by 2005, TURP represented only 39 % of surgical procedures for BPH, due to the combined effect of fewer prostatic operations and more minimally invasive procedures.

Monopolar TURP possesses excellent outcomes with the long-term (over 10 years) documented follow-up reported in several studies (Table 6.5). Thomas et al. retrospectively assessed 217 patients with a mean follow-up of 13 years and found a durable favorable symptomatic and urodynamic results in the vast majority of patients [44]. Mishriki et al. reported a prospective analysis in 113 evaluable patients and found a statistically significant improvement in QoL, bother scores, IPSS scores, and maximum flow rate at 12-year follow-up [45]. Masumori et al. demonstrated that IPSS and quality of life were still significantly better than baseline at 12 years follow-up, especially when preoperative urodynamic bladder outlet obstruction was confirmed [46]. These findings were mirrored by Hoekstra et al., who followed 150 men prospectively randomized between TURP, laser prostatectomy, and electrovaporization of the prostate, reporting 10-year actuarial failure rates of 0.11 for TURP, 0.22 for laser prostatectomy, and 0.23 for electrovaporization, whereas long-term peak flow results only remained significantly improved following TURP [47].

In another publication, Varkarakis et al. presented long-term morbidity of 577 patients with a minimum follow-up of 10 years [48]. They described an overall reintervention rate of 6 % and excellent functional outcomes. Noteworthy because of an impressive follow-up 12–22 years later are findings by Koshiba et al., who reported a reoperation rate of 5.6 % within this period [49].

Regarding the morbidity of TURP, Reich et al. analyzed 10,654 patients and found decreased mortality (0.1 %) and a morbidity that was lower than previous studies but remained at a significant level of 11.1 % [50]. The most relevant complications were failure to void (5.8 %), surgical revision (5.6 %), significant urinary tract infection (3.6 %), bleeding requiring transfusions (2.9 %), and transurethral

Table 6.4 Current guidelines recommendation on open prostatectomy, TURP, and TUIP

	OP	TURP	TUIP
EAU [4]	First choice of surgical treatment in men with drug-refractory LUTS secondary to BPO and prostate sizes >80–100 mL in the absence of holmium lasers (grade A)	Monopolar TURP is the current surgical standard procedure for men with prostate sizes of 30–80 mL and moderate to severe LUTS secondary to BPO. Monopolar TURP provides subjective and objective improvement rates superior to medical or minimally invasive treatments (grade A). Bipolar TURP achieves short-term results comparable to monopolar TURP (grade A)	Surgical therapy of choice for men with LUTS secondary to BPO and prostate sizes <30 mL without middle lobes (grade A)
AUA [6]	Option – for men with very enlarged prostate glands, may be more effective than TURP in relieving BOO, and for men with bladder diverticula/stones	TURP is an appropriate and effective primary alternative for surgical therapy in men with moderate to severe LUTS and/or who are significantly bothered by these symptoms. The choice of a monopolar or bipolar approach should be based on the patient's presentation, anatomy, the surgeon's experience, and discussion of the potential risks and likely benefits	Option – in men with moderate to severe LTS and/or who are significantly bothered by these symptoms when prostate size <30 ml
ICNDPCPD [41]	Acceptable	Acceptable	Not mentioned
CUA [42]	Option – for men whose prostates, in the view of the treating urologist, are too large for TURP	Monopolar TURP remains the gold standard treatment for patients with bothersome moderate or severe LUTS who request active treatment or who either fail or do not want medical therapy (grade B). Bipolar TURP has evolved as an equivalent alternative to the monopolar technique (grade B)	Option – for men with prostate gland volumes <30 g
JUA [5]	Associated with high incidence of complications but provides sustained efficacy, especially for large prostates (grade B)	TURP is the standard, most extensively performed surgical technique for the treatment of BPH. It is usually applicable to a BPH of up to moderate size (<50–80 mL)	It is applicable to relatively small-sized prostates (<20–30 mL) (grade B)

EAU European Association of Urology, *AUA* American Urological Association, *ICNDPCPD* International Consultation on New Developments in Prostate Cancer and Prostate Diseases, *CUA* Canadian Urological Association, *JUA* Japanese Urological Association

Table 6.5 TURP: long-term outcomes

References	No. of patients	Length of Follow-up, years	Main findings
Thomas	217	13	Significant sustained decrease in the majority of symptoms and improvements of urodynamic parameters.
			Long-term symptomatic failure and decreased flow rate principally associated with detrusor under activity rather than obstruction
Mishriki	113	12	Improvements in the QOL and bother scores were consistent and statistically significant
Masumori	34	12	Improved IPSS and QoL at 3 months gradually deteriorated with time, but patients at 12 years still significantly better than those at baseline
Hoekstra	29	10	IPSS, QoL, SPI, and BII still improved from values before treatment
			Only TURP group with long-term results of Q_{max} still improved
			10-year actuarial failure rate for TURP: 0.11 (CI 0.03–0.20)

resection syndrome (1.4 %). In another landmark study, Rassweiler et al. reported that the major late complications were urethral strictures (2.2–9.8 %) and bladder neck contractures (0.3–9.2 %), and the re-treatment rate was in the range 3–14.5 % after 5 years [51].

Bipolar electrosurgical technology for TURP has gained worldwide attention over the past 10 years with various companies introducing various devices [52, 53]. In contrast to monopolar systems such as TURP, bipolar energy systems use high-frequency electric current flowing between two electrodes within the surgical instrument to create a TURP-resection loop. The major advantage of bipolar energy systems is the use of saline as irrigation fluid, thus eliminating the risk of TUR syndrome [54].

Several RCTs have become available in the literature comparing standard (monopolar) TURP versus other surgical options for BPH (Table 6.6). Mamoulakis et al. published a meta-analysis on the head-to-head comparison between monopolar and bipolar TURP [55]. Sixteen RCTs published from 2004 to 2009 were included. No clinically relevant differences in short-term (12-months) efficacy were detected (Q_{max}: WMD: 0.72 ml/s; 95 % CI, 0.08–1.35; $p=0.03$). Treating 50 patients (95 % CI, 33–111) and 20 patients (95 % CI, 10–100) with bipolar TURP results in one fewer case of TUR syndrome (risk difference: 2.0 %; 95 % CI, 0.9–3.0 %; $p=0.01$) and one fewer case of clot retention (RD: 5.0 %; 95 % CI, 1.0–10 %; $p=0.03$), respectively. Operation times, transfusion rates, retention rates after catheter removal, and urethral complications did not differ significantly. Irrigation and catheterization duration was significantly longer with monopolar TURP (WMD: 8.75 h; 95 % CI, 6.8–10.7, and WMD: 21.77 h; 95 % CI, 19.22–24.32; $p<0.00001$,

Table 6.6 Monopolar TURP versus other treatment options: level 1 evidence

Reference	Study design	Patients, n	Comparator	Conclusions
Mamoulakis et al. [55]	Meta-analysis of 16 RCTs	1,406	B-TURP	No clinically relevant differences in short-term efficacy between the two techniques. No differences regarding OT and AEs. B-TURP better in terms of TUR syndrome and clot retention, as well as irrigation and catheterization time
Autorino et al. [56]	Single-center RCT	70		Clinical efficacy of bipolar TURP is comparable with that of monopolar TURP at 4-years follow-up
Mamoulakis et al. [57]	Multicenter RCT	279		Midterm (3-years) safety and efficacy of bipolar and monopolar TURP are comparable
Muslumanoglu et al. [58]	Single-center RCT	67		100 months results suggest that PlasmaKinetic technology can be used as a first-line treatment
Burke et al. [59]	Meta-analysis of 21 RCTs	1,936	B-TURP, PVP, HoLAP	Short-term advantages shown with bipolar TURP and PVP must be weighed against the long-term outcomes
Ahyai et al. [60]	Meta-analysis of 23 RCTs	2,245	B-TURP, B-TUVP, HoLEP, PVP	Statistically comparable efficacy and overall morbidity for MISTs versus contemporary TURP

TURP transurethral resection of the prostate, *B-TURP* bipolar transurethral resection of the prostate, *PVP* photoselective vaporization of the prostate, *HoLAP* holmium laser ablation of the prostate, *B-TUVP* bipolar transurethral vaporization of the prostate, *HoLEP* holmium laser enucleation of the prostate, *MISTs* minimally invasive surgical treatments

respectively). As various bipolar systems represent distinct technological advancements based on different electrophysiological principles regarding current flow, efficacy and safety concerns should be ideally separately evaluated for each system. When performing subgroup analyses, the authors did not observe any major effects on postoperative parameters among the systems evaluated in trials.

At the time of this meta-analysis, the authors also noted the limited follow-up available in the studies. Autorino et al. reported the first RCTs study to evaluate midterm (4-years) results of standard versus bipolar TURP [56]. Seventy patients with symptomatic BPH were enrolled. The significant improvements in both groups were maintained at 4 years for the IPSS, quality of life score, Q(max), and PVR versus baseline values. The main outcome variables at 4 years for bipolar and monopolar TURP were mean IPSS 6.9 and 6.4 ($p=0.58$); mean Q_{max} 19.8 ml/s and 21.2 ml/s ($p=0.44$), and mean PVR volume 42 ml and 45 ml ($p=0.3$). Overall, 2 of

32 (6.2 %) and 3 of 31 (9.6 %) patients required reoperation because of late complications ($p=0.15$). The major study limitation was the small sample size. More recently, an international multicenter RCT comparing bipolar with monopolar TURP was reported to compare the midterm safety/efficacy of the two techniques [57]. The bipolar TURP was performed by using the *AUTOCON II 400 electrosurgical unit* (Karl Storz, Tuttlingen, Germany). A total of 279 patients received treatment after allocation. Mean follow-up was 28.8 months, and a total of 186 of 279 patients (66.7 %) completed the 36-month follow-up. Ten urethral strictures cases were seen in each arm (monopolar TURP vs. bipolar TURP: 9.3 % vs. 8.2 %; $p=0.959$). Two versus eight bladder neck contracture cases (monopolar TURP vs. bipolar TURP: 1.9 % vs. 6.6 %; $p=0.108$) were collectively detected. Efficacy was similar between arms and durable. A total of 10 of 230 patients (4.3 %) experienced failure to cure and needed re-intervention without significant differences between arms.

A longer follow-up was reported by Muslumanoglu et al. who analyzed 67 patients (34 in the bipolar and 33 in the standard TURP group) who completed the 100-month follow-up [58]. IPSS increased to 8.5 ± 1.6 and 9.4 ± 0.9 in the bipolar group and 7.9 ± 1.3 and 8.7 ± 1.2 in the TURP group at 60 and 100 months, respectively. Mean maximal flow rate increased to 17.2 ± 3.9 mL/s in the bipolar group and to 16.9 ± 4.1 mL/s at 12 months in the TURP group but decreased to 15.9 ± 2.5 and 15.8 ± 3.0, respectively ($p=0.34$), at 100 months.

In another meta-analysis study, Burke et al. performed a systematic review of the published data from 21 RCTs evaluating photoselective vaporization of the prostate (PVP), holmium laser ablation (HoLAP), or bipolar TURP compared with monopolar TURP for the surgical treatment of BPO. Of these three emerging technologies, bipolar TURP was found to have the most RCT evidence available, with 81 % of the studies included in this review [59]. The authors concluded that surgical treatment with bipolar TURP resulted in similar improvement in symptom scores and urinary flow rates while reducing the duration of catheterization, hospitalization, and rates of clot retention. However, the short-term advantages shown with bipolar TURP and PVP must be weighed against the long-term outcomes of these procedures.

In another report, Ahyai et al. analyzed 20 contemporary RCTs published between 2005 and 2009 with an overall sample size of 954 TURP patients and a maximum follow-up of 5 years [60]. TURP resulted in a substantial improvement of mean Q_{max} (+162 %) and a significant reduction of mean IPSS (−70 %), mean QoL scores (−69 %), and mean post-void residual urine (0–77 %). This was also indirectly shown by a 45–65 % prostate-specific antigen (PSA) reduction. However, TURP and HoLEP seem to challenge the gold standard in terms of efficacy. The analysis also demonstrated that the diversity of possible complications after TURP, leading to an increased cumulative risk of adverse events. Most relevant complications include bleeding requiring blood transfusion (2 %; range: 0–9), TUR syndrome (0.8 %; range: 0–5), AUR (4.5 %; range: 0–13.3), clot retention (4.9 %; range: 0–39), and UTI (4.1 %; range: 0–22), and these findings are in agreement with those from other large analyses [50]. TURP was associated with the highest risk of bleeding with subsequent need for blood transfusion and remains the only procedure still carrying the risk of documented TUR syndrome. Nevertheless, the analysis also demonstrated that the overall morbidity of TURP is not statistically significantly different compared to minimally invasive procedures. This could be explained by the few late complications and the low long-term failure rate of TURP, as also suggested in the nationwide analysis of 20,671 patients reported by Madersbacher et al., showing a cumulative incidence of secondary procedures following a TURP of 2.9, 5.8, and 7.4 % at 1, 5, and 8 years, respectively [30].

TUIP (Transurethral Incision of the Prostate)

The transurethral incision of prostate (TUIP) was introduced by Orandi in the early 1970s, and it involves cutting the prostate at the 5 and 7 o'clock positions of the bladder neck to open the prostatic urethra without removal of prostate tissue [61, 62]. This procedure represents an apparently simpler, less costly, and less invasive treatment option than TURP for men with small (<30 ml) prostate glands, and it can be eventually performed under local anesthesia [63].

Two systematic reviews have been reported so far, comparing TUIP with TURP. In 2001, Yang et al. identified and analyzed 9 RCTs involving a total of 691 participants randomized to TUIP ($n=346$) or TURP ($n=345$) [64]. Generally patients were included only if they had a relatively small prostate (<30 g). Statistically and potentially clinically significant differences were in favor of TURP for maximum urinary flow rate, but no differences were evident for symptoms recorded. TUIP was found to have several advantages over TURP, including a lower incidence of complications (20 % vs. 31 %), fewer blood transfusions (0.9 % vs. 25.1 %), decreased risk of retrograde ejaculation (21 % vs. 73 %), and shorter operative time (20 min difference) and hospital stay (mean 4.4–6.2 days for TUIP and 4.4–8.4 days for TURP). In addition, the treatments had equivalent postoperative catheterization duration and reoperation rate within the first 12 months.

More recently, Lourenco et al. also reported a systematic review and meta-analysis of short and long-term data from RCTs comparing TUIP with TURP [65]. Compared to Yang et al. [64], they identified two additional studies, and overall they included data from 795 participants with mainly mild to moderate BPE across 10 RCTs. Again, no clear evidence of superiority emerged on meta-analysis regarding primary outcome of improvement in symptom score at 12 months. In contrast, TURP was clearly superior in terms of urodynamic improvement with a consistent and statistically significant greater increase in peak urinary flow rate. Thus, the authors speculated that men with mild to moderate of BPE would be content with the symptom improvement gained with TUIP. On the other hand, TUIP did demonstrate further advantages in terms of reduced comorbidity and hospitalization, with blood transfusion rates significantly lower with TUIP (11 % vs. 28). However, it should be noted that subjects recruited for these trials were all treated prior to 1991, and equipment, perioperative care, and training for urologists performing TURP have dramatically improved over the past 20 years. TUIP did not show advantage in terms of reducing the risk of longer-term adverse effects such as urinary incontinence, erectile dysfunction, or stricture formation although reporting of these events was inconsistent. Meta-analysis confirmed lower rates of ejaculatory dysfunction following TUIP with a 50 % risk reduction (27.6 % vs. 51.8 %), and this could represent an important issue for sexually active men with isolated bladder neck hypertrophy.

In terms of treatment cost, TUIP shows benefit in terms of reducing operating time (18.9 min shorter) and hospital stay (−2.26 days), but this must be balanced by the higher rate of reoperation in the longer term (TUIP 18.4 % vs. TURP 7.2 %), a finding in contrast to Yang et al. [64]. Both meta-analyses concluded that ideally an adequately powered, multicenter RCT comparing TUIP and TURP should be performed, but this is unlikely given the advancement of other technologies such as laser energy together with the long follow-up required to assess reoperation rate [64, 65].

Current guidelines still maintain a role for TUIP in selected cases, i.e., patients with small (<30 ml) glands (Table 6.4) [4–6, 41, 42].

Other Options Based on Bipolar Technology (TUERP and TURisV)

The transurethral enucleation and resection of the prostate (TUERP) in patients using the PlasmaKinetic™ system was recently reported by Liu et al., who assessed the results obtained in 1,100 patients [66]. As in open prostatectomy, in TUERP the resectoscope tip mimics the tip of the surgeon index finger to detach the en bloc lobes from the surgical capsule and enable true anatomical enucleation of a prostate of any size. Mean follow-up was 4.3 years. Mean preoperative prostate weight was 67.7 g (range 35–256). Mean catheter time was 1.8 days and mean hospital stay was 5.3 days. Significant, pronounced, immediate, and lasting improvement in the IPSS, maximum urinary flow, and post-void residual urine volume was obtained. There were few postoperative complications, such as urinary tract infection, urethral stricture, meatal stenosis, and bladder neck contracture, in all patients, and the transfusion rate was 0.8 %.

Reich et al. recently published initial clinical results of bipolar plasma vaporization of the prostate with a mushroomlike electrode from Olympus [67]. The rationale for this feasibility study was based on the introduction of a new device with a similar safety and efficacy profile as lasers but at substantially lower costs. Despite the promising results, the authors recognized the limitations of this study to be the small sample (30 patients), the lack of a comparative arm, and the short follow-up (only 6 months). Isotani et al. later reported their experience with this innovative endoscopic surgical modality, defined as TURisV [68]. They performed 17 cases with a median volume of vaporized prostate tissue of 41.1 g. No changes in hemoglobin or electrolyte levels were seen postoperatively, and good outcomes were obtained, suggesting that the procedure is safe and efficacious.

Conclusions

Given the widespread use of medical therapies and the introduction of a myriad of minimally invasive treatments, the patient population undergoing the most traditional and established procedures for BPO, such as open simple prostatectomy and TURP, has considerably changed over the last two decades. Overall, available evidence suggests that good long-term outcomes can be obtained with both surgical options, with TURP being still considered the gold standard treatment. Simple prostatectomy still has a role in certain instances and also appears to be safe and efficacious options in contemporary series, especially in settings where more recent (laser) technology is not available. TUIP can be still regarded as a viable option in selected patient with a suitable (small) gland.

Improvements in instrumentation, surgical technique, irrigation fluids, antibiotics, and anesthesia have made the modern TURP a safe operation. The most relevant innovation over the last years has been represented by the bipolar systems, which has minimized the morbidity of conventional TURP. As we are facing older patients presenting with more comorbidities, with a longer history of medical therapy for BPH and larger prostates, it is likely for bipolar TURP to play a major role, which will be supported by accumulating data on its long-term efficacy.

Recently introduced technologies, such as TUERP and TURisV, seem promising and user-friendly, but further clinical investigation is needed to define their role in the surgical armamentarium for BPO.

References

1. Vela-Navarrete R, et al. The impact of medical therapy on surgery for benign prostatic hyperplasia: a study comparing changes in a decade (1992–2002). BJU Int. 2005;96:1045–8.
2. Izard J, Nickel JC. Impact of medical therapy on transurethral resection of the prostate: two decades of change. BJU Int. 2011;108(1):89–93.
3. Takeuchi M, Masumori N, Tsukamoto T. Contemporary patients with LUTS/BPH requiring prostatectomy have long-term history of treatment with alpha1-blockers and large prostates compared with past cases. Urology. 2009;74(3):606–9.
4. Madersbacher S, Alivizatos G, Nordling J, Sanz CR, Emberton M, de la Rosette JJ. EAU 2004 guidelines on assessment, therapy and follow-up of men with lower urinary tract symptoms suggestive of benign prostatic obstruction (BPH guidelines). Eur Urol. 2004;46(5):547–54.
5. Homma Y, Gotoh M, Yokoyama O, et al. Outline of JUA clinical guidelines for benign prostatic hyperplasia. Int J Urol. 2011;18(11):741–56.
6. McVary KT, Roehrborn CG, Avins AL, et al. Update on AUA guideline on the management of benign prostatic hyperplasia. J Urol. 2011;185(5):1793–803.
7. Fuller E. Six successful and successive cases of prostatectomy. J Cut Genitourin Dis. 1895;13:229.
8. McGill AF. Suprapubic prostatectomy. Br Med J. 1887;2:1104.
9. Freyer PJ. Total extirpation of the prostate for radical cure of enlargement of that organ (with four successful cases). Br Med J. 1901;2:125–9.
10. Freyer PJ. One thousand cases of total enucleation of the prostate for radical cure of enlargement of that organ. Br Med J. 1912;2:869–70.

11. Millin T. Retropubic prostatectomy: a new extravesical prostatectomy. Report on 20 cases. Lancet. 1945;246:693–6.
12. Macalister C, Kelly PM, Millin T. Retropubic prostatectomy. Experiences based on 757 cases. Lancet. 1949;253:381–5.
13. Young HH. VIII. Conservative perineal prostatectomy: the results of two years' experience and report of seventy-five cases. Ann Surg. 1905;41(4):549–57.
14. Bruskewitz R. Management of symptomatic BPH in the US: who is treated and how? Eur Urol. 1999;36 suppl 3:7–13.
15. Lukacs B. Management of symptomatic BPH in France: who is treated and how? Eur Urol. 1999;36 suppl 3:14–20.
16. Ahlstrand C, Carlsson P, Jonsson B. An estimate of the life-time cost of surgical treatment of patients with benign prostatic hyperplasia in Sweden. Scand J Urol Nephrol. 1996;30: 37–43.
17. Serretta V, Morgia G, Fondacaro L, Members of the Sicilian-Calabrian Society of Urology, et al. Open prostatectomy for benign prostatic enlargement in southern Europe in the late 1990s: a contemporary series of 1800 interventions. Urology. 2002;60:623–7.
18. Mozes B, Cohen YC, Olmer L, et al. Factors affecting change in quality of life after prostatectomy for benign prostatic hypertrophy: the impact of surgical techniques. J Urol. 1996;155: 191–6.
19. Masumori N, Kamoto T, Seki N, Homma Y, Committee for Clinical Guideline for Benign Prostatic Hyperplasia. Surgical procedures for benign prostatic hyperplasia: a nationwide survey in Japan. Int J Urol. 2011;18(2):166–70.
20. Servadio C. Is open prostatectomy really obsolete? Urology. 1992;40(5):419–21.
21. Bernie JE, Schmidt JD. Simple perineal prostatectomy: lessons learned from a modern series. J Urol. 2003;170(1):115–8.
22. Meier DE, Tarpley JL, Imediegwu OO, et al. The outcome of suprapubic prostatectomy: a contemporary series in the developing world. Urology. 1995;46(1):40–4.
23. Condie Jr JD, Cutherell L, Mian A. Suprapubic prostatectomy for benign prostatic hyperplasia in rural Asia: 200 consecutive cases. Urology. 1999;54(6):1012–6.
24. Tubaro A, Carter S, Hind A, Vicentini C, Miano L. A prospective study of the safety and efficacy of suprapubic transvesical prostatectomy in patients with benign prostatic hyperplasia. J Urol. 2001;166(1):172–6.
25. Varkarakis I, Kyriakakis Z, Delis A, Protogerou V, Deliveliotis C. Long-term results of open transvesical prostatectomy from a contemporary series of patients. Urology. 2004;64(2): 306–10.
26. Adam C, Hofstetter A, Deubner J, et al. Retropubic transvesical prostatectomy for significant prostatic enlargement must remain a standard part of urology training. Scand J Urol Nephrol. 2004;38(6):472–6.
27. Helfand B, Mouli S, Dedhia R, McVary KT. Management of lower urinary tract symptoms secondary to benign prostatic hyperplasia with open prostatectomy: results of a contemporary series. J Urol. 2006;176(6 Pt 1):2557–61.
28. Gratzke C, Schlenker B, Seitz M, et al. Complications and early postoperative outcome after open prostatectomy in patients with benign prostatic enlargement: results of a prospective multicenter study. J Urol. 2007;177(4):1419–22.
29. Suer E, Gokce I, Yaman O, Anafarta K, Göğüş O. Open prostatectomy is still a valid option for large prostates: a high-volume, single-center experience. Urology. 2008;72(1):90–4.
30. Madersbacher S, Lackner J, Brössner C, et al. Reoperation, myocardial infarction and mortality after transurethral and open prostatectomy: a nation-wide, long-term analysis of 23,123 cases. Eur Urol. 2005;47(4):499–504.
31. Gregoir W. Haemostatic prostatic adenomectomy. Eur Urol. 1978;4(1):1–8.
32. Walsh PC, Oesterling JE. Improved hemostasis during simple retropubic prostatectomy. J Urol. 1990;143(6):1203–4.
33. Amen-Palma JA, Arteaga RB. Hemostatic technique: extracapsular prostatic adenomectomy. J Urol. 2001;166:1364–7.

34. Srougi M, Dall'Oglio MF, Bomfim AC, Andreoni C, Cury J, Ortiz V. An improved technique for controlling bleeding during simple retropubic prostatectomy. BJU Int. 2003;92(7):813–7.
35. Dall'Oglio MF, Srougi M, Antunes AA, Crippa A, Cury J. An improved technique for controlling bleeding during simple retropubic prostatectomy: a randomized controlled study. BJU Int. 2006;98(2):384–7.
36. Shaheen A, Quinlan D. Feasibility of open simple prostatectomy with early vascular control. BJU Int. 2004;93(3):349–52.
37. Djaladat H, Mehrsai A, Saraji A, Moosavi S, Djaladat Y, Pourmand G. Suprapubic prostatectomy with a novel catheter. J Urol. 2006;175(6):2083–6.
38. Okorie CO, Salia M, Liu P, Pisters LL. Modified suprapubic prostatectomy without irrigation is safe. Urology. 2010;75(3):701–5.
39. Simforoosh N, Abdi H, Kashi AH, et al. Open prostatectomy versus transurethral resection of the prostate, where are we standing in the new era? A randomized controlled trial. Urol J. 2010;7(4):262–9.
40. Ou R, You M, Tang P, Chen H, Deng X, Xie K. A randomized trial of transvesical prostatectomy versus transurethral resection of the prostate for prostate greater than 80 mL. Urology. 2010;76(4):958–61.
41. Abrams P, Chapple C, Khoury S, Roehrborn C, de la Rosette J. International consultation on new developments in prostate cancer and prostate diseases. Evaluation and treatment of lower urinary tract symptoms in older men. J Urol. 2013;189(1 Suppl):S93–101.
42. Nickel JC, Méndez-Probst CE, Whelan TF, Paterson RF, Razvi H. 2010 update: guidelines for the management of benign prostatic hyperplasia. Can Urol Assoc J. 2010;4(5):310–6.
43. Hawtrey CE, Williams RD. Historical evolution of transurethral resection at the University of Iowa: Alcock and Flocks. J Urol. 2008;180(1):55–61.
44. Thomas AW, Cannon A, Bartlett E, et al. The natural history of lower urinary tract dysfunction in men: minimum 10-year urodynamic follow-up of transurethral resection of prostate for bladder outlet obstruction. J Urol. 2005;174(5):1887–91.
45. Mishriki SF, Grimsley SJ, Nabi G, et al. Improved quality of life and enhanced satisfaction after TURP: prospective 12-year follow-up study. Urology. 2008;72(2):322–6.
46. Masumori N, Furuya R, Tanaka Y, et al. The 12-year symptomatic outcome of transurethral resection of the prostate for patients with lower urinary tract symptoms suggestive of benign prostatic obstruction compared to the urodynamic findings before surgery. BJU Int. 2010;105:1429–33.
47. Hoekstra RJ, Van Melick HH, Kok ET, et al. A 10-year follow-up after transurethral resection of the prostate, contact laser prostatectomy and electrovaporization in men with benign prostatic hyperplasia; long-term results of a randomized controlled trial. BJU Int. 2010;106(6):822–6.
48. Varkarakis J, Bartsch G, Horninger W. Long-term morbidity and mortality of transurethral prostatectomy: a 10- year follow-up. Prostate. 2004;58:248–51.
49. Koshiba K, Egawa S, Ohori M, Uchida T, Yokoyama E, Shoji K. Does transurethral resection of the prostate pose a risk to life? 22-year outcome. J Urol. 1995;153:1506–9.
50. Reich O, Gratzke C, Bachmann A, et al. Morbidity, mortality and early outcome of transurethral resection of the prostate: a prospective multicenter evaluation of 10,654 patients. J Urol. 2008;180(1):246–9.
51. Rassweiler J, Teber D, Kuntz R, Hofmann R. Complications of transurethral resection of the prostate (TURP)–incidence, management, and prevention. Eur Urol. 2006;50(5):969–79.
52. Ubee SS, Philip J, Nair M. Bipolar technology for transurethral prostatectomy. Expert Rev Med Devices. 2011;8(2):149–54.
53. Rassweiler J, Schulze M, Stock C, Teber D, De La Rosette J. Bipolar transurethral resection of the prostate–technical modifications and early clinical experience. Minim Invasive Ther Allied Technol. 2007;16(1):11–21.
54. Hawary A, Mukhtar K, Sinclair A, Pearce I. Transurethral resection of the prostate syndrome: almost gone but not forgotten. J Endourol. 2009;23(12):2013–20.

55. Mamoulakis C, Ubbink DT, de la Rosette JJ. Bipolar versus monopolar transurethral resection of the prostate: a systematic review and meta-analysis of randomized controlled trials. Eur Urol. 2009;56(5):798–809.
56. Autorino R, Damiano R, Di Lorenzo G, et al. Four-year outcome of a prospective randomised trial comparing bipolar plasmakinetic and monopolar transurethral resection of the prostate. Eur Urol. 2009;55(4):922–9.
57. Mamoulakis C, Schulze M, Skolarikos A, et al. Midterm results from an international multi-centre randomised controlled trial comparing bipolar with monopolar transurethral resection of the prostate. Eur Urol. 2013;63(4):667–76.
58. Muslumanoglu AY, Yuruk E, Binbay M, Akman T. Transurethral resection of prostate with plasmakinetic energy: 100 months results of a prospective randomized trial. BJU Int. 2012;110(4):546–9.
59. Burke N, Whelan JP, Goeree L, et al. Systematic review and meta-analysis of transurethral resection of the prostate versus minimally invasive procedures for the treatment of benign prostatic obstruction. Urology. 2010;75(5):1015–22.
60. Ahyai SA, Gilling P, Kaplan SA, et al. Meta-analysis of functional outcomes and complications following transurethral procedures for lower urinary tract symptoms resulting from benign prostatic enlargement. Eur Urol. 2010;58(3):384–97.
61. Orandi A. Transurethral incision of the prostate. J Urol. 1973;110:229–31.
62. Orandi A. Transurethral resection versus transurethral incision of the prostate. Urol Clin North Am. 1990;17:601–12.
63. Irani I, Bon D, Fournier F, Doré B, Aubert J. Patient acceptability of transurethral incision of the prostate under local anaesthesia. Br J Urol. 1996;78(6):904–6.
64. Yang Q, Peters TJ, Donovan JL, Wilt TJ, Abrams P. Transurethral incision compared with transurethral resection of the prostate for bladder outlet obstruction: a systematic review and meta-analysis of randomized controlled trials. J Urol. 2001;165(5):1526–32.
65. Lourenco T, Shaw M, Fraser C, MacLennan G, N'Dow J, Pickard R. The clinical effectiveness of transurethral incision of the prostate: a systematic review of randomised controlled trials. World J Urol. 2010;28(1):23–32.
66. Liu C, Zheng S, Li H, Xu K. Transurethral enucleation and resection of prostate in patients with benign prostatic hyperplasia by plasma kinetics. J Urol. 2010;184(6):2440–5.
67. Reich O, Schlenker B, Gratzke C, et al. Plasma vaporisation of the prostate: initial clinical results. Eur Urol. 2010;57(4):693–7.
68. Isotani S, Muto S, Yu J, et al. Clinical and safety profiles of bipolar transurethral vaporization of the prostate in saline: a preliminary report. Asian J Endosc Surg. 2012;5(1):21–4.

Chapter 7
Surgical Treatment: Lasers and Techniques

Sascha A. Ahyai, Andreas Becker, Malte Rieken, and Alexander Bachmann

Abstract Laser techniques for the treatment of benign prostate enlargement are established alternatives to TURP and OP. Currently, the most frequently used lasers are holmium (Ho):YAG, potassium titanyl phosphate or lithium triborate (GreenLight), thulium, and diode laser. Based on the wavelength of the laser and the resulting laser–tissue interaction enucleation, vaporization, vapoenucleation, and vaporesection are the main techniques. In recent years, high-level evidence could show the equal efficacy and superior safety of holmium laser enucleation of the prostate (HoLEP) to TURP and OP. Furthermore, photoselective vaporization of the prostate (PVP) demonstrated comparable efficacy and superior safety in comparison to TURP and OP in various randomized clinical trials (RCTs). Thulium and diode laser prostatectomy represent upcoming new techniques with promising results. Although, short- and intermediate-term results indicate comparable outcomes relative to TURP or HoLEP, long-term results are missing and more high-level evidence results are required. Diode lasers, primarily used for vaporization, are characterized by high intraoperative safety. Controversial data exist regarding postoperative complications and reoperation rate of diode lasers.

Keywords Holmium laser enucleation • Laser vaporization • Lower urinary tract symptoms • Minimally invasive therapy • Benign prostate enlargement • Surgical therapy

---

S.A. Ahyai • A. Becker (✉)
Department of Urology, University Medical Center Hamburg,
Martinistraße 52, Hamburg 20246, Germany
e-mail: sahyai@uke.de; a.becker@uke.de

M. Rieken, MD • A. Bachmann, MD
Department of Urology, University Hospital Basel,
Spitalstr. 21, Basel 4031, Switzerland

Introduction

Historically, it was Einstein in 1917 who discovered the concept of focused beams of coherent light and stimulated emission of microwaves and hereby introduced the physical principals of laser. The term laser, invented by Gould in 1957, is an acronym and stands for "light amplification by stimulated emission of radiation". Three years later, in 1960, Maiman produced the first rubin laser. Parson and Mulvaney were the first urologists who tested the rubin laser experimentally (1966) and clinically (1968).

Laserlight consists of a single wavelength (monochromatic) of coherent light. The energy of this light will be converted into warmth respectively heat when it is absorbed. In a surgical setting, there are normally two ways of laser–tissue interaction that are being used: coagulation (with temperatures below) and vaporization (with temperatures above the boiling point). The extent of tissue ablation is defined by the rate of the applied energy, which again depends on the wavelength of the laser (Table 7.1). Furthermore, the operating modus "pulsed" or "continuous" wave also influences the power and tissue penetration of the laser. For this reason, one needs to know, that laser does not mean laser. Each laser has its specific wavelength, absorbing medium, and penetration depth.

Holmium Laser Enucleation of the Prostate

Background

Initially, the Ho:YAG laser was used in terms of a holmium laser resection of the prostate (HoLRP) introduced by Gilling und Fraundorfer in 1996 [30]. Two years later a tissue morcellator was introduced making a Holmium laser enucleation of the prostate (HoLEP) possible [32]. Since then HoLEP was investigated in multiple randomized trials [16, 33, 45, 47, 55, 56] and represents today the most rigorously analyzed laser prostatectomy [3].

Equipment and Surgical Technique

Equipment

We use the 100 W Holmium laser power suite (VersaPulse, Lumenis, Yokneam, Israel) to perform HoLEP (Fig. 7.1). Filter protection glasses and a camera-based video system are mandatory to provide optical safety for involved staff and the patient. The outer sheet of a continuous flow transurethral resection system (26 French) is used with a modified inner sheet containing a laser bridge. An end-fire

Table 7.1 RCTs comparing laser techniques to TURP or OP – key parameters and main results

Author	System	Comparator	Follow-up (months)	Number of patients	Main results
Al-Ansari et al. [5]	PVP (120 W HPS)	TURP	36	120	Operation time shorter with TURP Significantly higher transfusion rate with TURP Comparable functional results Higher reoperation rate after TURP
Bouchier-Hayes et al. [13]	PVP (80 W KTP)	TURP	12	120	Shorter duration of catheterization and hospitalization after PVP Comparable functional results Less bleeding complications after TURP
Capitan et al. [15]	PVP (120 W HPS)	TURP	24	100	Shorter duration of catheterization and hospitalization after PVP Comparable functional results
Horasanli et al. [43]	PVP (80 W KTP)	TURP	6	76	Operation time shorter with TURP Functional results after TURP superior to PVP
Lukacs et al. [49]	PVP (120 W HPS)	TURP	12	139	Non-inferiority of PVP regarding IPSS-reduction could not be shown Other functional results comparable
Pereira-Correia et al. [60]	PVP (120 W HPS)	TURP	24	20	Comparable improvement of urodynamic parameters in both groups
Skolarikos et al. [70]	PVP (80 W KTP)	OP	18	125	Shorter operating time with OP Significantly higher transfusion rate after OP Improvement of QoL after OP superior to PVP
Gilling et al. [34]	HoLEP	TURP	84	120	HoLEP is at least equivalent to TURP in the long term with fewer reoperations being necessary
Ahyai et al. [4]	HoLEP	TURP	36	200	HoLEP resulted in significantly better micturition parameters and less perioperative morbidity
Montorsi et al. [55]	HoLEP	TURP	12	100	Similar effectiveness and complication rate after HoLEP and TURP. HoLEP associated with shorter catheterization time and hospital stay

(continued)

Table 7.1 (continued)

Author	System	Comparator	Follow-up (months)	Number of patients	Main results
Eltabey et al. [24]	HoLEP	TURP	12	80	Shorter catheterization times, hospital stays, lower hemoglobin loss, and greater improvement of voiding function after HoLEP compared to TURP
Mavuduru et al. [53]	HoLEP	TURP	9	30	Comparative effectiveness and safety with the advantage of reduced intraoperative hemorrhage and perioperative morbidity
Chen et al. [16]	HoLEP	Bipolar TURP	24	280	HoLEP: less risk of hemorrhage, decreased bladder irrigation and catheter times, reduced hospital stay
Kuntz et al. [46]	HoLEP	OP	60	120	HoLEP and OP equally effective for removal of large prostatic adenomas. Less perioperative morbidity after HoLEP
Naspro et al. [56]	HoLEP	OP	24	80	Similar functional results 2 years after HoLEP or OP. Reduced catheterization, hospital stay, and blood loss after HoLEP
Xia et al. [81]	ThuVARP	TURP	12	100	Superior safety and equivalent efficacy compared to TURP for small- and medium-size prostates
Peng et al. [59]	ThuVARP	Bipolar TURP	3	100	Superior safety and equivalent efficacy at 3 months after ThuVARP compared to bipolar TURP
Zhang et al. [82]	ThuLEP	HoLEP	18	133	Comparable safety and efficacy of ThuLEP and HoLEP

7 Surgical Treatment: Lasers and Techniques

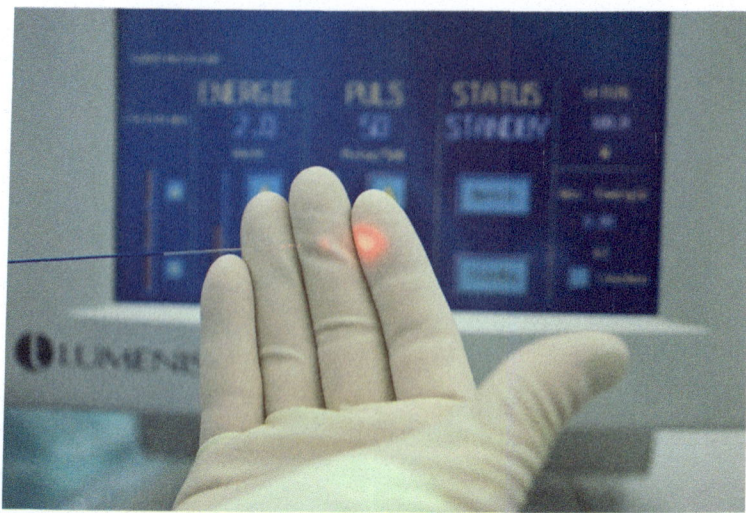

Fig. 7.1 End-fire laser fiber and Holmium laser power suite, 100 W (VersaPulse, Lumenis, Yokneam, Israel) (Photo: Axel Kirchhof/UKE)

laser fiber is advanced, guided by a 7 French tube, until the fiber end protrudes the tip of the resectoscope. To remove enucleated tissue from the bladder, a morcellation device is needed. As no electric energy is applied, isotonic saline solution is used as irrigation fluid.

Surgical Technique

Traditionally, as described by Gilling et al. [31] as a first step, the laser is used to make two incisions from the lip of the bladder neck at 5 and 7 o'clock to the verumontanum (three-lobe technique, Fig. 7.2a). These incisions are deepened to the surgical capsule, which is optically identified. Subsequently, a third horizontal incision just in front of the verumontanum connects the apical ends of the first incisions. Gently lifting the middle lobe with the shaft of the laser resectoscope, the laser fiber follows the anatomical plain between prostatic tissue and the surgical capsule until the lip of the bladder neck is reached and the retrograde enucleation of the middle lobe is completed (Fig. 7.2b). Detaching the remaining tissue from the bladder can float into the bladder. As a second step, the bottom edges of the side lobes are incised with semicircular incisions following the surgical capsule from 5 to 7 o'clock position. Due to the hemostatic effect of the holmium laser, blood vessels are usually immediately sealed during the incision. Accordingly, this step is repeated starting from a 12 o'clock at the upper part of the side lobes. Subsequently, the side lobes are dissected extending them laterally and following the capsule until the bladder neck is reached and the side lobe

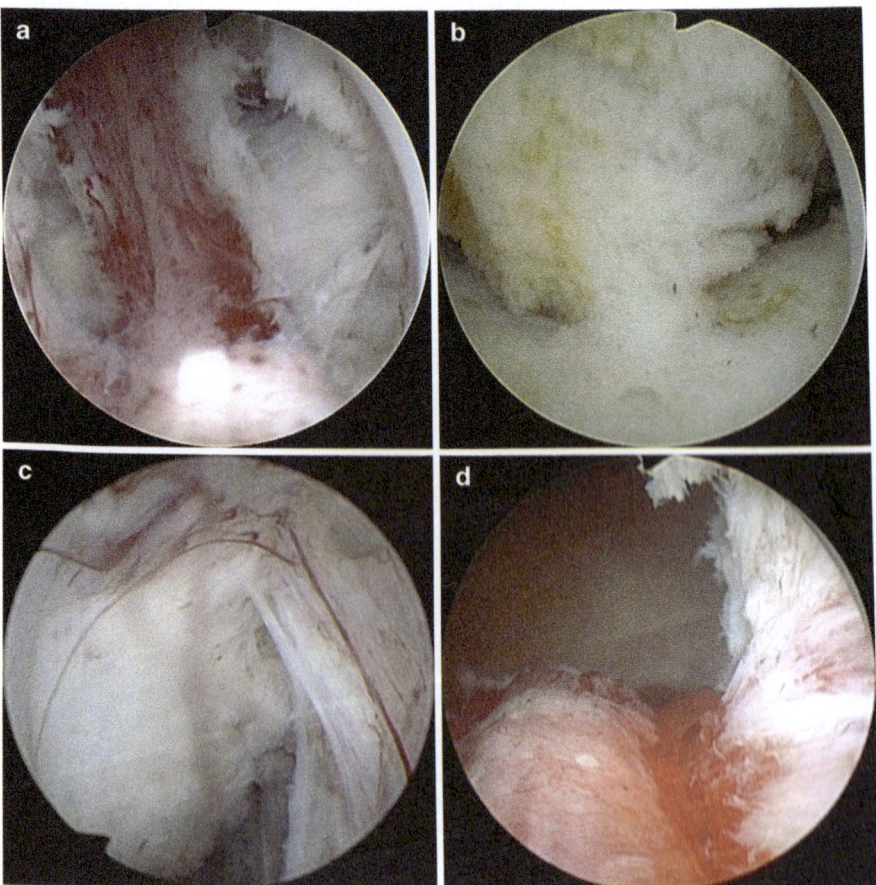

Fig. 7.2 Holmium laser enucleation as initially described by Gilling et al. [31]: incisions of the bladder neck at 5 and 7 o'clock to the verumontanum (**a**). Enucleation of the middle lobe, connecting the 5 and 7 o'clock incisions following the anatomical plains between prostatic tissue and the surgical capsule until the lip of the bladder neck is reached. The middle lobe remains detached by a small bridge of mucosa (**b**). Subsequently, the bottom edges of the side lobes are mobilized with semicircular incisions following the surgical capsule, starting at 6 o'clock position (**c**). This step is accordingly repeated starting from a 12 o'clock position, mobilizing the upper part of the side lobes. Subsequently, the lower and the upper incisions are connected extending them laterally and following the surgical capsule until the lip of the bladder neck is reached and the side lobe again is pushed in the lumen of the bladder. After having completed this step for both side lobes, the prostate channel is wide (**d**) (Photo: S. Ahyai)

again is pushed in the lumen of the bladder. After having completed this step for both side lobes, the prostate channel is wide, offering clear view to the smooth face of the surgical capsule (Fig. 7.2d). The defocused laser is used to c minor bleedings from the capsule. As a last step, the tissue floating in the bladder has to be removed using a morcellation device. Sucki tip of a morcellator, a small blade rapidly cuts the tissue. The

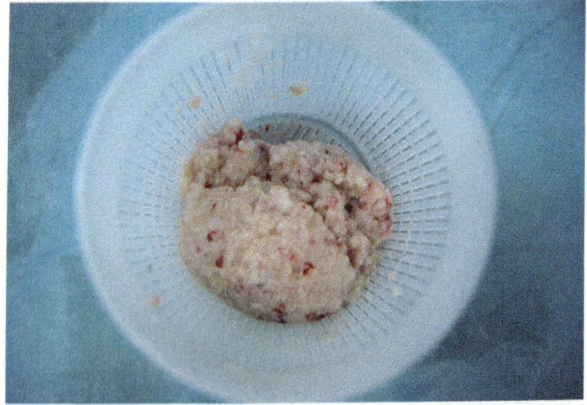

Fig. 7.3 HoLEP specimen after morcellation (Photo: S. Ahyai)

prostate are suctioned through the morcellator into a collector, allowing complete histopathologic examination of the specimen (Fig. 7.3). During the morcellation process, it is necessary to keep the bladder lumen filled with fluid, to prevent injury of the bladder wall. After evacuation of remaining blood clots, a 20 French 3-way catheter, allowing further irrigation, should be placed.

Meanwhile we adapted our operating technique according to the presence of a middle lobe, size, shape of the prostate itself, and finally the angle between prostate and bladder. If there is no middle lobe, we perform only one incision at 5 o'clock to separate the prostate into left and right (two-lobe technique). If the angle between prostate and bladder is very steep, a deep bladder neck incision at 5 and 7 o'clock remains crucial (even if there is no middle lobe) to prevent undermining of the bladder neck during retrograde enucleation of the side lobes. If the prostate is not too big and the angle towards the bladder rather shallow, enucleation of the whole prostate in one piece is possible commencing at the verumontanum with the left apical lobe ("one-lobe" technique). In contradistinction to the traditional technique, we found enucleation of the side lobes generally more comfortable when turning the instrument upside down after the surgical plane is found (Fig. 7.4). Furthermore, our lateral mobilization of the side lobes is continued up to 12 o'clock. By this means the lobes are only attached to a small bridge of mucosa and tissue, when the anterior commissure is incised (Fig. 7.5).

Indications and Outcomes

comparable efficacy and a lower complication rate for HoLEP compared to proven in a total of 8 RCTs [14, 33, 37, 45, 53, 65, 77, 80]. They low intra- and perioperative morbidity, statistically significater catheter time, shorter hospital stay, and similar shortional outcome, compared to TURP (Table 7.2). A recent LEP as the only minimally invasive LUTS treatment

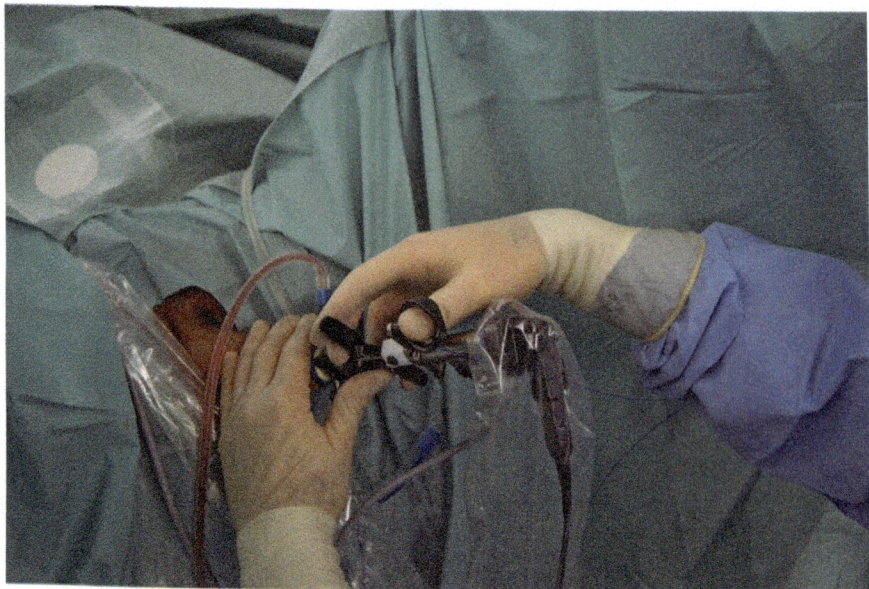

Fig. 7.4 Modified upside-down enucleation of the side lobes (Photo: S. Ahyai)

Fig. 7.5 Modified preparation of the side lobes: continuing the 6 o'clock incision to 12 o'clock position and omitting a second incision at 12 o'clock, side lobes remain attached to a small bridge of mucosa and tissue, until the anterior commissure is incised (Photo: S. Ahyai)

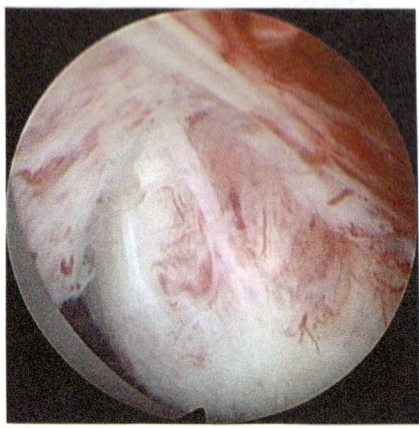

that provides a more pronounced reduction of voiding-related symptoms and increase of urinary flow rate after HoLEP compared to TURP [3]. Possibly, the complete enucleation of the prostatic (obstructing) tissue, resulting in a wide prostatic cavity, similar to OP, provides superior and more durable voiding function compared to other ablative procedures. As PSA represents a surrogate for prostate volume in BPH patients, a reported mean PSA drop of >80 % after HoLEP further underlines the substantial removal of prostatic tissue [71].

Although, overall intra- and postoperative complication rate seems to be c rable, postoperative urgency seems to be slightly higher in HoLEP p

7 Surgical Treatment: Lasers and Techniques

Table 7.2 Comparison of selected laser prostatectomy techniques

Technique/parameter	Holmium laser enucleation of the prostate	Photoselective vaporization of the prostate	Thulium laser prostatectomy	Diode laser prostatectomy
Operative technique	Enucleation	Vaporization	Vaporization, Enucleation, Vaporesection, Vapoenucleation	Vaporization, Enucleation
Fiber	Front-firing	Side-firing	Front-firing	Side-firing, Front-firing, Contact mode
Wavelengths	2,000 nm	532 nm	2,000 nm	940 nm, 980 nm, 1,318 nm, 1,470 nm
RCTs vs. TURP	Yes	Yes	Yes	No
RCTs vs. OP	Yes	Yes	No	No
Safety in patients with anticoagulation	Yes	Yes	Yes	Yes
Longest follow-up case series	6 years	5 years	1 year	1 year
Longest follow-up RCTs	7 years	3 years	18 months	NA

occurs in 5.6 and 2.2 % of cases after HoLEP and TURP, respectively [55, 56]. We believe that it is generally important to inform patients who undergo prostate surgery that urgency can occur postoperatively, but is mostly self-limiting and transient [55]. However, persistent stress urinary incontinence is rarely reported (<1 %) and seems to occur in a similar frequency as after TURP [62]. In their most recent follow-up at 7 years after HoLEP or TURP, respectively, Gilling and colleagues report no differences considering voiding parameters like urinary flow rate and AUA score, as well as sexual function- and voiding function-related quality of life scores. Typical late complications after HoLEP are similar to other transurethral procedures and include bladder neck stenosis (0–3 %), urethral strictures (2–8 %), and urinary stress incontinence (0–3 %) [3].

Compared to OP, which is considered as the reference standard of surgical treatment for prostates with a volume of more than 80–100 ml [50, 58], HoLEP showed lower perioperative complications, statistically significantly reduced blood loss, lower transfusion rates, as well as a shorter catheterization time and hospital stay in two randomized controlled trials (Table 7.2) [46, 56]. Short- and intermediate-time functional results (international prostate symptom score, residual urine, urinary flow rate) after 1, 3, and 6 months were comparable to those after open surgery. Follow-up results up to 5–7 years after randomization of participants of the RCTs have been published and confirm the comparability of functional results after HoLEP compared to OP [47] and TURP [34], all providing excellent voiding function and a low rate of late complications [29, 34, 47]. Compared to OP, HoLEP seems to provide virtually identical functional results at 5 years after surgery [47].

In both groups a comparable low rate of reoperations (OP: 6.7 vs. HoLEP: 5.0 %, $P=1.0$) and no BPH recurrence were reported.

The physical characteristics of the Holmium laser enable a precise incision of prostatic tissues with a simultaneous coagulation of vessels to a depth of 2–3 mm, providing excellent hemostatic properties. Accordingly, HoLEP has been applied to patients otherwise unfit for surgical intervention. For example, Elzayat and colleagues reported about feasibility of HoLEP in patients on anticoagulation therapy [25]. Although transfusion rate was elevated (10 %), they reported no major bleeding or thromboembolic complications in their comorbid cohort of patients. In another recent retrospective study, 39 patients on oral anticoagulation (33 % with Coumadin) were compared to a control group not undergoing anticoagulation therapy. Interestingly, they found no differences in bleeding complications between the groups, none of the patients requiring blood transfusion [75]. Within our institutional database (2006–2010) 73 of 631 (11.3 %) patients (37 and 63 % of them on platelet inhibition and low molecular weight heparin therapy, respectively) underwent HoLEP under anticoagulation therapy. In this cohort of patients, bleeding complications were more frequent compared to the control group (platelet inhibitor, 15 % vs. heparin, 15 % vs. control, 5 %, $p=0.002$). However, severe complications (GIII) were rarely recorded and occurred in a similar frequency in patients with platelet and heparin anticoagulation compared to no anticoagulation patients (4 % vs. 7 % vs. 2 %, $p=0.097$) (unpublished data).

Due to the widespread use of PSA testing, the risk of being diagnosed with incidental PCa after surgery for BPE decreased from 23 to 7 % for T1a and from 15 to 2 % for T1b [74]. Although most of these patients might have insignificant disease, up to 21 % are at risk for clinical progression [21]. Concerns have been raised that laser-based treatment alternatives with a high amount of vaporization (e.g., photoselective vaporization, diode laser vaporization, thulium/YAG vaporesection) may limit or disable histopathological diagnosis, particularly for patients with a life expectancy of more than 10 years. However, unlike most other laser technologies, vaporization during HoLEP is minimal and histopathologic evaluation of virtually all removed tissue is possible.

Even after a rigorous prostate cancer screening at our institution, suggesting saturation biopsy after 2 sets of negative 12-core biopsies in the case of suspicious PSA level, the rate of incidental prostate cancer after HoLEP was as high as 11 % (A. Becker, S.A. Ahyai, 2012, unpublished data). Of the patients aged 70 or less, 69 % underwent non-curative treatment (active surveillance or androgen deprivation therapy), 5 % underwent radiation therapy, and 26 % were scheduled for radical prostatectomy, revealing localized (pT2c) stage and Gleason pattern 3+4 in all but one patient with vanishing tumor. These results underline the importance of collecting and processing tissue during LUTS surgery in younger patients.

Palliative TURP is associated with a significant proportion of treatment failure and incontinence [51] and worse functional results compared to TURP in BPO patients [20]. Therefore, even more than in BPH there seems to be a demand for alternative effective and less invasive surgical procedures than pTURP. Up to date, no evidence-based data regarding the feasibility of HoLEP in such patients is available. Our institutional data, including 62 patients with known prostate cancer who underwent HoLEP, suggest that palliative HoLEP might be a feasible, save, and effective treatment option. As complication rate, even in combination with a subsequent radiotherapy, seems very acceptable (5 % complications GIII), palliative HoLEP might not be just a palliative procedure but also a step in a multimodal treatment concept in patients with LUTS and prostate cancer [12].

Potential Drawbacks and Complications

One main finding of the RCTs comparing HoLEP and TURP/OP was a consistently longer operative time for HoLEP compared to TURP (mean: +20 min) or even OP (mean: +40 min) [45, 46]. However, those studies represented the early era of HoLEP when mechanical tissue morcellators [32], which increase the speed of HoLEP, were not available and the prostatic lobes were fragmented with an electrocautery loop after having been enucleated subtotally. Particularly in large prostates, this so-called mushroom technique [41] is time-consuming. In matched pair analysis of contemporary patients managed with either HoLEP, TURP, or OP, tissue retrieval rate and operating time in HoLEP were significantly faster compared to TURP and similar to OP [2].

Regarding the advantages HoLEP provides compared to TURP, open prostatectomy, and other minimally invasive treatment approaches, one wonders why HoLEP has not already replaced TURP and OP all over the world as the new gold standard for the treatment of LUTS, as many prominent authors postulate [6, 27, 76]. One thing that probably shunned many urologic surgeons from adopting HoLEP in their clinical practice is that for surgeons trained on transurethral resection, technique and laser equipment used for HoLEP seem not to be very intuitive. Therefore, anatomical enucleation of the prostate using a technically complex laser approach represents a challenge for every HoLEP learner.

However, intraoperative vision during HoLEP is improved due to less bleeding and a prolonged operative time does not expose the patient to the risk of TUR syndrome. Several publications on the learning curve of HoLEP imply that, similar to other surgical procedures, a number of at least 20 procedures seem necessary to become familiar with the technique [22, 69]. During the learning curve, complications like transient urgency and urinary incontinency are more prevalent [1, 22]. However, incidence decreases after approximately 50 procedures [61]. General recommendations include being endoscopically skilled, starting with prostates of moderate size [39], and, ideally, performing the first procedures under supervision of an experienced mentor. Given these conditions, HoLEP seems to provide durable results and a low rate of complications and reoperation, even during the learning process [26].

Urge and Stress Incontinence: Urinary incontinence remains one of the major risks and drawbacks of any LUTS procedure. Concerns have raised that the rate of stress and urge incontinence after HoLEP might be as high as 35 and 9 %, respectively [1]. Indeed, irritative voiding symptoms (dysuria, urge) are constantly reported for 10–70 % of all patients during the early postoperative period and seem to be more pronounced after HoLEP than after TURP [27, 56, 58, 65]. However, this condition has been shown to be transient and self-limiting in most cases [1, 27, 55], and the true rate of persistent incontinence after HoLEP seems to vary between 1 and 3 % [3, 55].

Erectile dysfunction (ED) and LUTS represent two common medical conditions that seem to be associated with each other due to anatomic and hormonal changes in aging men [48, 66]. However, the impact of LUTS surgery has been controversially discussed over the last decades, and a contemporary sub-analysis of RCT comparing HoLEP and TURP implied that neither HoLEP nor TURP showed a detrimental effect on erectile function [14]. Specifically, at a 24-month follow-up, the authors recorded a slightly nonsignificant improvement of erectile function compared to baseline in both groups. Nevertheless, orgasmic function was affected by retrograde ejaculation in 77 and 78 %, after TURP and HoLEP, respectively, and patients should be informed extensively.

Summary

- HoLEP is a safe and effective treatment alternative to TURP and OP.
- The short- and long-term functional results are comparable to TURP and OP.
- HoLEP is superior to TURP and OP with regard to perioperative safety.
- HoLEP has demonstrated a superior cost-effectiveness compared to TURP and OP.

Photoselective Vaporization of the Prostate (PVP)

Background

Photoselective vaporization with the GreenLight laser evolved from visual laser ablation of the prostate (VLAP) with the 1,064 nm neodymium–yttrium–aluminum–garnet (Nd:YAG) laser which was introduced in the early 1990s [19]. Due to the low absorption coefficient and a penetration depth of 4–18 mm, a deep coagulative necrosis was observed in most tissues [44]. Despite an advantageous intraoperative safety profile, the functional outcome was inferior to TURP. Furthermore, a high reoperation rate was observed so that VLAP has been abandoned [42, 78].

The advent of the potassium titanyl phosphate (KTP) laser can be regarded as the renaissance of laser techniques in prostate surgery. When passing the Nd:YAG-produced laser beam (1,046 nm) through a KTP crystal, the frequency is doubled and the wavelength halved. The resulting wavelength of 532 nm is in the range of visible green light. This gives the laser also the name GreenLight laser. The light produced by the GreenLight laser has a completely different laser beam–tissue interaction than the Nd:YAG laser. The wavelength is not absorbed by water but strongly absorbed by hemoglobin. This results in enhanced hemostatic properties. The absorption depth in vascularized tissue as in the prostate is only 1–3 mm. This generates a high energy density. The high energy density in the prostate tissue leads to a rapid vaporization of the water in the tissue. Because of this effect, the technique is also called photoselective vaporization of the prostate (PVP) [54, 72].

A widespread use of the technique was achieved with the introduction of the 80 W KTP laser (American Medical Systems Inc., Minnetonka, MN, USA). Since 2007, the 120 W high performance system (HPS) laser (American Medical Systems Inc., Minnetonka, MN, USA) has been on the market. The HPS laser is equipped with a lithium triborate (LBO) crystal and a fiber that produces a more collimated laser beam. The 180 W accelerated power system (XPS) laser (American Medical Systems Inc., Minnetonka, MN, USA) was brought onto the market in 2010. Despite its 50 % increase in power, the 180 W laser is equipped with a liquid cooled fiber that can emit a higher amount of energy [10, 11]. Furthermore, the area of the laser beam is increased by 50 % in comparison to the 120 W laser. The increase in laser beam area results in faster tissue vaporization [63].

Equipment and Surgical Technique

Equipment

The equipment necessary for PVP consists of the laser generator and the single-use laser fiber, which is introduced in a specific laser cystoscope. The laser cystoscope allows separation of the laser fiber and the saline irrigation solution. The laser fiber of PVP uses a so-called side-firing technique. This means that the laser beam leaves the fiber on the side and not on the tip of the fiber. Tissue can be vaporized under direct vision. The recommended distance between prostate surface and laser fiber is about 1 mm. This provides an optimal energy delivery to the tissue and a maximum vaporization effect. Tissue vaporization is demonstrated by formation of visible bubbles. If bleeding occurs, increasing the tissue fiber distance to 3 mm can induce coagulation.

Surgical Technique

As with TURP, several techniques of PVP have been described. In contrast to TURP, the main movement of tissue ablation is not in forward and backward direction but by a side sweeping of the laser fiber beam. The fiber is slowly rotated between the thumb and the index finger and moved anterior and posterior. The overall goal of PVP is to achieve a nonobstructive prostatic urethra that has a smooth tissue surface. The surgeon should develop an approach that is efficient, safe, and reproducible. At our center, the so-called Basel technique is performed [35]. This surgical technique consists of various steps. First, an anterior working space is created to avoid the contact of the fiber with the tissue and to create a connection between the bladder and the apex. Once that channel has been created, the lateral lobes are vaporized between the bladder neck and the apex by sweeping the fiber laterally. After that, the apical tissue and the median lobe are ablated and the bladder neck is opened. The median lobe is always treated at the end of the procedure, because tissue contact and subsequent fiber degradation occurs more frequently at the median lobe. Treating the median lobe last avoids early fiber degradation, which is especially important when treating large prostates. At the end of the procedure, a TURP-like cavity should have been created. Finally, hemostasis is controlled and coagulation is performed where necessary. At the end of the procedure, a catheter is inserted and, according to center, preoperative retention and size of the prostate kept between just a few hours and a few days.

Indications and Outcomes

The indications for PVP are comparable with the indications for TURP. Surgery is usually required when the patient experiences recurrent or refractory urinary retention, overflow incontinence, bladder stones, recurrent urinary tract infection, or recurrent gross hematuria due to prostate enlargement or dilatation of the upper urinary tract due to benign prostate enlargement. Furthermore, progressive symptoms under conservative treatment are an indication for surgery. For virtually all patients with an indication for TURP, PVP is a possible treatment alternative. In addition to TURP, other groups of patients can also be safely operated with PVP. Due to the hemostatic properties of PVP, patients with increased surgical risk of bleeding like bleeding disorders or on-going oral anticoagulation or platelet aggregation inhibition are eligible for PVP. Furthermore, prostates >80 ml can effectively be treated with PVP.

PVP leads to a rapid and durable improvement of voiding parameters and micturition symptoms. Currently, data with a maximum follow-up of 5 years are available. In a single-center study of 500 patients, the improvement of voiding parameters (IPSS/QoL) and micturition symptoms (maximum flow rate, postvoid residual volume) remained statistically significant throughout the follow-up period of 5 years. No difference between patients with and without increased risk of bleeding could be detected regarding perioperative and postoperative parameters [67]. Similar results are reported from a single-surgeon series with an improvement of IPSS by 79 %, QoL by 80 %, maximum flow rate by 172 %, and postvoid residual volume by 77 %, respectively [38].

Various prospective randomized trials (RCTs) compared PVP with the 80 and 120 W laser to TURP [10, 11]. Table 7.1 summarizes results of recent RCTs comparing PVP and TURP. On average, operating time was by around 20 min longer with PVP than with TURP. Duration of catheterization and hospitalization could be reduced by on average of 2 days with PVP, respectively. Improvement of IPSS, maximum flow rate, and postvoid residual volume was comparable between both techniques in six studies, whereas in one study PVP was superior and in two studies patients in the TURP arm achieved superior results [73]. No significant difference regarding erectile function and sexual satisfaction could be detected between both techniques during a 1-year follow-up [49]. Furthermore, comparable urodynamic desobstruction can be achieved with either technique [49].

When comparing PVP with the 80 W laser to open prostatectomy (OP) in patients with a prostate volume >80 ml, operating time is significantly longer with PVP by 30 min on average, whereas duration of catheterization and hospitalization is significantly reduced. The improvement of maximum flow rate and postvoid residual volume is comparable after 18-month follow-up, whereas the reduction of QoL score and prostate volume was significantly higher in the OP arm [70]. PVP demonstrated to achieve a significantly improvement of voiding parameters and symptoms in patients with a prostate volume >120 ml [79]. Compared to HoLEP in patients with a prostate volume >60 ml operating time was comparable with 80 W PVP. However, the improvements of maximum flow rate, postvoid residual volume, PSA value, and prostate volume were significantly higher in the HoLEP group [23].

Potential Drawbacks and Complications

The intraoperative and postoperative safety on PVP could be demonstrated in various studies.

When comparing TURP in PVP in RCTs, the rate of perioperative blood transfusions is significantly less with PVP (0.3 % vs. 6.9 %, $p=0.003$). A meta-analysis of all available RCTs ($n=7$) found no significant difference between PVP and TURP regarding the incidence of postoperative retention, urinary tract infection, gross hematuria, or incidence of urethral strictures, or bladder neck contractures [73]. Compared to OP, the transfusion rate with PVP is significantly less (0 % vs. 13.3 %), whereas the reoperation rate after a follow-up of 18 months was comparable [70].

The hemostatic properties of PVP make it ideal for the application in patients with increased risk of bleeding. Patient can continue their oral anticoagulation or platelet aggregation inhibition perioperatively. In a study of 162 patients under warfarin (19 %), ASS (62 %), clopidogrel (12 %), or 2 or more anticoagulants (7 %), except one case of severe fluid retention, no intraoperative complication occurred. In the first 30 postoperative days, 4 % of patients suffered from bleeding, 2 % needed a blood transfusion, and a surgical revision was indicated in 1 % [18].

Summary

- PVP is a safe and effective treatment alternative to TURP.
- The short- and midterm functional results are comparable to TURP.

- PVP is superior to TURP with regard to perioperative safety.
- PVP can safely be performed in patients with increased perioperative risk.

Upcoming Laser Techniques

Besides the two most established and commonly used techniques – which are represented by HoLEP and PVP – several alternative laser techniques are currently in the phase of clinical and scientific evaluation. Of those, the thulium–yttrium–aluminum–garnet (Tm:YAG) laser has been investigated, including evidence from two randomized controlled trials (Table 7.2) [59, 81], and found consideration in the most recent EAU guidelines [57]. The physical characteristics of the Tm:YAG laser allow rapid vaporization as well as smooth incision of the prostatic tissue (Table 7.1) [7]. Accordingly, the thulium laser is currently applied in different approaches, using either enucleation technique (ThuLEP) [9], vaporization techniques (ThuVaP) [52], or techniques combining both principles such as vaporesection (ThuVARP) [81] or vapoenucleation (ThuVEP) [36].

As intraoperative safety of ThuVARP has been demonstrated in two RCTs [59, 81], ThuVARP is recommended as an alternative to TURP in small- and medium-sized prostates [57]. Moreover, evidence from case series indicates intraoperative safety of ThuVEP in patients on anticoagulative therapy [40] or with larger prostates [8]. Although short- and intermediate-time functional results after ThuLEP seem comparable to those after HoLEP [82], to date, no long-term follow-up is available for any Tm:YAG laser approach. In general, although high-level evidence for thulium laser prostatectomy is available, the quantity and quality of trials – with a total of 3 RCTs, overall including 311 patients with a follow-up of respectively 3, 12, and 18 months, are inferior compared to PVP or HoLEP (Table 7.1). Furthermore, comparison of thulium laser prostatectomy with the current gold standards (TURP, OP, HoLEP) is hampered by the diversity of surgical approaches and different techniques (ThuLEP, ThuVAP, ThuVARP, ThuVEP) (Table 7.2).

Diode lasers represent another promising laser technique. The light of diode lasers is generated by semiconductors. The wavelength depends on the semiconductor used (Table 7.2). The main advantage of diode lasers compared to Nd:YAG lasers are a much smaller laser generator size. Furthermore, diode lasers work energy efficient and therefore can be operated from a standard power outlet. It is important to notice that there exists no diode laser per se. Wavelength, power output, pulse generation, and fiber design influence laser–tissue interaction. Thus, energy density and penetration depth vary strongly between different wavelengths and even between different models of the same wavelength. Tissue necrosis induced by diode laser application ranges from 1.3 to 4.5 mm in ex vivo models. In canine experiments, a necrotic zone of 6.1 mm was observed [64]. In comparison, the necrotic zone with PVP is around 1.5 mm.

In principle, two techniques – diode laser vaporization of the prostate (DLVP) and diode laser enucleation of the prostate (DiLEP) – are currently applied in the context of surgical treatment of LUTS. The surgical technique of DLVP resembles that of PVP, whereas DiLEP is comparable to other enucleating techniques like HoLEP.

DLVP leads to a rapid and significant improvement of voiding parameters and micturition symptoms. In two prospective comparable trials between PVP with the 120 W laser and DLVP with a 200 W 980 nm diode laser, comparable functional results regarding improvement of voiding parameters (IPSS, QoL) and micturition symptoms (maximum flow rate, postvoid residual volume) could be achieved [17, 68]. Comparable postoperative functional results with significant improvement of all relevant parameters are reported from cohort studies with a 120 W 980 nm diode laser and a 150 W 980 nm diode lasers [28].

Due to the limited number of studies, the lack of results beyond a follow-up of 1 year and the lack of RCTs in comparison to TURP or OP currently no clear recommendation for the application of diode lasers outside clinical trials can be given.

Summary

- Thulium and diode lasers represent promising alternative laser techniques and are currently in the phase of clinical and scientific evaluation.
- The thulium laser is applied in different approaches, using either enucleation technique (ThuLEP), vaporization techniques (ThuVaP), or techniques combining both principles such as vaporesection (ThuVARP) or vapoenucleation (ThuVEP).
- Various laser types and techniques are available for diode laser prostatectomy.
- Short– and intermediate-term outcomes comparable to TURP or HoLEP have been demonstrated on high evidence level for thulium laser prostatectomy (ThuVARP and ThuLEP).
- Long-term efficacy of thulium laser prostatectomy has not yet been confirmed.
- Diode laser prostatectomy can safely be performed in patients with increased perioperative risk.
- Currently no intermediate- and long-term data are available and no recommendation for the diode laser prostatectomy outside clinical trials can be given.

References

1. Abdel-Hakim AM, Habib EI, et al. Holmium laser enucleation of the prostate: initial report of the first 230 Egyptian cases performed in a single center. Urology. 2010;76(2):448–52.
2. Ahyai SA, Chun FK, et al. Transurethral holmium laser enucleation versus transurethral resection of the prostate and simple open prostatectomy – which procedure is faster? J Urol. 2012;187(5):1608–13.
3. Ahyai SA, Gilling P, et al. Meta-analysis of functional outcomes and complications following transurethral procedures for lower urinary tract symptoms resulting from benign prostatic enlargement. Eur Urol. 2010;58(3):384–97.

4. Ahyai SA, Lehrich K, et al. Holmium laser enucleation versus transurethral resection of the prostate: 3-year follow-up results of a randomized clinical trial. Eur Urol. 2007;52(5):1456–63.
5. Al-Ansari A, Younes N, et al. GreenLight HPS 120-W laser vaporization versus transurethral resection of the prostate for treatment of benign prostatic hyperplasia: a randomized clinical trial with midterm follow-up. Eur Urol. 2010;58(3):349–55.
6. Alivizatos G, Skolarikos A. Should holmium laser enucleation be the new gold standard for bladder outlet obstruction caused by BPH? Nat Clin Pract Urol. 2008;5(7):358–9.
7. Bach T, Muschter R, et al. Laser treatment of benign prostatic obstruction: basics and physical differences. Eur Urol. 2012;61(2):317–25.
8. Bach T, Netsch C, et al. Thulium:YAG vapoenucleation in large volume prostates. J Urol. 2011;186(6):2323–7.
9. Bach T, Xia SJ, et al. Thulium: YAG 2 mum cw laser prostatectomy: where do we stand? World J Urol. 2010;28(2):163–8.
10. Bachmann A, Muir GH, et al. 180-W XPS GreenLight laser therapy for benign prostate hyperplasia: early safety, efficacy, and perioperative outcome after 201 procedures. Eur Urol. 2012;61(3):600–7.
11. Bachmann A, Woo HH, et al. Laser prostatectomy of lower urinary tract symptoms due to benign prostate enlargement: a critical review of evidence. Curr Opin Urol. 2012;22(1):22–33.
12. Becker A, et al. Holmium laser enucleation of the prostate is safe in patients with prostate cancer and lower urinary tract symptoms – a retrospective feasibility study. J Endourol (in press).
13. Bouchier-Hayes DM, Van Appledorn S, et al. A randomized trial of photoselective vaporization of the prostate using the 80-W potassium-titanyl-phosphate laser vs transurethral prostatectomy, with a 1-year follow-up. BJU Int. 2010;105(7):964–9.
14. Briganti A, Naspro R, et al. Impact on sexual function of holmium laser enucleation versus transurethral resection of the prostate: results of a prospective, 2-center, randomized trial. J Urol. 2006;175(5):1817–21.
15. Capitan C, Blazquez C, et al. GreenLight HPS 120-W laser vaporization versus transurethral resection of the prostate for the treatment of lower urinary tract symptoms due to benign prostatic hyperplasia: a randomized clinical trial with 2-year follow-up. Eur Urol. 2011;60(4):734–9.
16. Chen YB, Chen Q, et al. A prospective, randomized clinical trial comparing plasmakinetic resection of the prostate with holmium laser enucleation of the prostate based on a 2-year follow-up. J Urol. 2013;189:217–22.
17. Chiang PH, Chen CH, et al. GreenLight HPS laser 120-W versus diode laser 200-W vaporization of the prostate: comparative clinical experience. Lasers Surg Med. 2010;42(7):624–9.
18. Chung DE, Wysock JS, et al. Outcomes and complications after 532 nm laser prostatectomy in anticoagulated patients with benign prostatic hyperplasia. J Urol. 2011;186(3):977–81.
19. Costello AJ, Johnson DE, et al. Nd:YAG laser ablation of the prostate as a treatment for benign prostatic hypertrophy. Lasers Surg Med. 1992;12(2):121–4.
20. Crain DS, Amling CL, et al. Palliative transurethral prostate resection for bladder outlet obstruction in patients with locally advanced prostate cancer. J Urol. 2004;171(2 Pt 1):668–71.
21. Descazeaud A, Peyromaure M, et al. Predictive factors for progression in patients with clinical stage T1a prostate cancer in the PSA era. Eur Urol. 2008;53(2):355–61.
22. El-Hakim A, Elhilali MM. Holmium laser enucleation of the prostate can be taught: the first learning experience. BJU Int. 2002;90(9):863–9.
23. Elmansy H, Baazeem A, et al. Holmium laser enucleation versus photoselective vaporization for prostatic adenoma greater than 60 ml: preliminary results of a prospective, randomized clinical trial. J Urol. 2012;188(1):216–21.
24. Eltabey MA, Sherif H, et al. Holmium laser enucleation versus transurethral resection of the prostate. Can J Urol. 2010;17(6):5447–52.

25. Elzayat E, Habib E, et al. Holmium laser enucleation of the prostate in patients on anticoagulant therapy or with bleeding disorders. J Urol. 2006;175(4):1428–32.
26. Elzayat EA, Elhilali MM. Holmium laser enucleation of the prostate (HoLEP): long-term results, reoperation rate, and possible impact of the learning curve. Eur Urol. 2007;52(5):1465–71.
27. Elzayat EA, Habib EI, et al. Holmium laser enucleation of the prostate: a size-independent new "gold standard". Urology. 2005;66(5 Suppl):108–13.
28. Erol A, Cam K, et al. High power diode laser vaporization of the prostate: preliminary results for benign prostatic hyperplasia. J Urol. 2009;182(3):1078–82.
29. Gilling PJ, Aho TF, et al. Holmium laser enucleation of the prostate: results at 6 years. Eur Urol. 2008;53(4):744–9.
30. Gilling PJ, Cass CB, et al. The use of the holmium laser in the treatment of benign prostatic hyperplasia. J Endourol. 1996;10(5):459–61.
31. Gilling PJ, Fraundorfer MR. Holmium laser prostatectomy: a technique in evolution. Curr Opin Urol. 1998;8(1):11–5.
32. Gilling PJ, Kennett K, et al. Holmium laser enucleation of the prostate (HoLEP) combined with transurethral tissue morcellation: an update on the early clinical experience. J Endourol. 1998;12(5):457–9.
33. Gilling PJ, Mackey M, et al. Holmium laser versus transurethral resection of the prostate: a randomized prospective trial with 1-year follow-up. J Urol. 1999;162(5):1640–4.
34. Gilling PJ, Wilson LC, et al. Long-term results of a randomized trial comparing holmium laser enucleation of the prostate and transurethral resection of the prostate: results at 7 years. BJU Int. 2012;109(3):408–11.
35. Gomez Sancha F, Bachmann A, et al. Photoselective vaporization of the prostate (GreenLight PV): lessons learnt after 3500 procedures. Prostate Cancer Prostatic Dis. 2007;10(4):316–22.
36. Gross AJ, Netsch C, et al. Complications and early postoperative outcome in 1080 patients after thulium vapoenucleation of the prostate: results at a single institution. Eur Urol. 2013;63(5):859–67.
37. Gupta N, Sivaramakrishna, et al. Comparison of standard transurethral resection, transurethral vapour resection and holmium laser enucleation of the prostate for managing benign prostatic hyperplasia of >40 g. BJU Int. 2006;97(1):85–9.
38. Hai MA. Photoselective vaporization of prostate: five-year outcomes of entire clinic patient population. Urology. 2009;73(4):807–10.
39. Haraguchi T, Takenaka A, et al. The relationship between the reproducibility of holmium laser enucleation of the prostate and prostate size over the learning curve. Prostate Cancer Prostatic Dis. 2009;12(3):281–4.
40. Hauser S, Rogenhofer S, et al. Thulium laser (Revolix) vapoenucleation of the prostate is a safe procedure in patients with an increased risk of hemorrhage. Urol Int. 2012;88(4):390–4.
41. Hochreiter WW, Thalmann GN, et al. Holmium laser enucleation of the prostate combined with electrocautery resection: the mushroom technique. J Urol. 2002;168(4 Pt 1):1470–4.
42. Hoffman RM, MacDonald R, et al. Laser prostatectomy versus transurethral resection for treating benign prostatic obstruction: a systematic review. J Urol. 2003;169(1):210–5.
43. Horasanli K, Silay MS, et al. Photoselective potassium titanyl phosphate (KTP) laser vaporization versus transurethral resection of the prostate for prostates larger than 70 mL: a short-term prospective randomized trial. Urology. 2008;71(2):247–51.
44. Kuntz RM. Current role of lasers in the treatment of benign prostatic hyperplasia (BPH). Eur Urol. 2006;49(6):961–9.
45. Kuntz RM, Ahyai S, et al. Transurethral holmium laser enucleation of the prostate versus transurethral electrocautery resection of the prostate: a randomized prospective trial in 200 patients. J Urol. 2004;172(3):1012–6.
46. Kuntz RM, Lehrich K. Transurethral holmium laser enucleation versus transvesical open enucleation for prostate adenoma greater than 100 gm.: a randomized prospective trial of 120 patients. J Urol. 2002;168(4 Pt 1):1465–9.

47. Kuntz RM, Lehrich K, et al. Holmium laser enucleation of the prostate versus open prostatectomy for prostates greater than 100 grams: 5-year follow-up results of a randomised clinical trial. Eur Urol. 2008;53(1):160–6.
48. Leliefeld HH, Stoevelaar HJ, et al. Sexual function before and after various treatments for symptomatic benign prostatic hyperplasia. BJU Int. 2002;89(3):208–13.
49. Lukacs B, Loeffler J, et al. Photoselective vaporization of the prostate with GreenLight 120-W laser compared with monopolar transurethral resection of the prostate: a multicenter randomized controlled trial. Eur Urol. 2012;61(6):1165–73.
50. Madersbacher S, Alivizatos G, et al. EAU 2004 guidelines on assessment, therapy and follow-up of men with lower urinary tract symptoms suggestive of benign prostatic obstruction (BPH guidelines). Eur Urol. 2004;46(5):547–54.
51. Marszalek M, Ponholzer A, et al. Palliative transurethral resection of the prostate: functional outcome and impact on survival. BJU Int. 2007;99(1):56–9.
52. Mattioli S, Munoz R, et al. Treatment of benign prostatic hyperplasia with the Revolix laser. Arch Esp Urol. 2008;61(9):1037–43.
53. Mavuduru RM, Mandal AK, et al. Comparison of HoLEP and TURP in terms of efficacy in the early postoperative period and perioperative morbidity. Urol Int. 2009;82(2):130–5.
54. McAllister WJ, Gilling PJ. Vaporization of the prostate. Curr Opin Urol. 2004;14(1):31–4.
55. Montorsi F, Naspro R, et al. Holmium laser enucleation versus transurethral resection of the prostate: results from a 2-center, prospective, randomized trial in patients with obstructive benign prostatic hyperplasia. J Urol. 2004;172(5 Pt 1):1926–9.
56. Naspro R, Suardi N, et al. Holmium laser enucleation of the prostate versus open prostatectomy for prostates >70 g: 24-month follow-up. Eur Urol. 2006;50(3):563–8.
57. Oelke M, Bachmann A, et al. EAU guidelines on the treatment and follow-up of non-neurogenic male lower urinary tract symptoms including benign prostatic obstruction. Eur Urol. 2013;64:118–40.
58. Ou R, You M, et al. A randomized trial of transvesical prostatectomy versus transurethral resection of the prostate for prostate greater than 80 mL. Urology. 2010;76(4):958–61.
59. Peng B, Wang GC, et al. A comparative study of thulium laser resection of the prostate and bipolar transurethral plasmakinetic prostatectomy for treating benign prostatic hyperplasia. BJU Int. 2013;111(4):633–7.
60. Pereira-Correia JA, de Moraes Sousa KD, et al. GreenLight HPS 120-W laser vaporization vs transurethral resection of the prostate (<60 mL): a 2-year randomized double-blind prospective urodynamic investigation. BJU Int. 2012;110(8):1184–9.
61. Placer J, Gelabert-Mas A, et al. Holmium laser enucleation of prostate: outcome and complications of self-taught learning curve. Urology. 2009;73(5):1042–8.
62. Rassweiler J, Teber D, et al. Complications of transurethral resection of the prostate (TURP) – incidence, management, and prevention. Eur Urol. 2006;50(5):969–79; discussion 980.
63. Rieken M, Bonkat G, et al. The effect of increased maximum power output on perioperative and early postoperative outcome in photoselective vaporization of the prostate. Lasers Surg Med. 2013;45(1):28–33.
64. Rieken M, Kang HW, et al. Laser vaporization of the prostate in vivo: experience with the 150-W 980-nm diode laser in living canines. Lasers Surg Med. 2010;42(8):736–42.
65. Rigatti L, Naspro R, et al. Urodynamics after TURP and HoLEP in urodynamically obstructed patients: are there any differences at 1 year of follow-up? Urology. 2006;67(6):1193–8.
66. Rosen R, Altwein J, et al. Lower urinary tract symptoms and male sexual dysfunction: the multinational survey of the aging male (MSAM-7). Eur Urol. 2003;44(6):637–49.
67. Ruszat R, Seitz M, et al. GreenLight laser vaporization of the prostate: single-center experience and long-term results after 500 procedures. Eur Urol. 2008;54(4):893–901.
68. Ruszat R, Seitz M, et al. Prospective single-centre comparison of 120-W diode-pumped solid-state high-intensity system laser vaporization of the prostate and 200-W high-intensive diode-laser ablation of the prostate for treating benign prostatic hyperplasia. BJU Int. 2009;104(6):820–5.

69. Santos Garcia-Baquero A, Soler Martinez J, et al. Prostatic enucleation with holmium laser. Arch Esp Urol. 2008;61(9):1015–21.
70. Skolarikos A, Papachristou C, et al. Eighteen-month results of a randomized prospective study comparing transurethral photoselective vaporization with transvesical open enucleation for prostatic adenomas greater than 80 cc. J Endourol. 2008;22(10):2333–40.
71. Tan AH, Gilling PJ, et al. A randomized trial comparing holmium laser enucleation of the prostate with transurethral resection of the prostate for the treatment of bladder outlet obstruction secondary to benign prostatic hyperplasia in large glands (40 to 200 grams). J Urol. 2003;170(4 Pt 1):1270–4.
72. Te AE. The development of laser prostatectomy. BJU Int. 2004;93(3):262–5.
73. Thangasamy IA, Chalasani V, et al. Photoselective vaporisation of the prostate using 80-W and 120-W laser versus transurethral resection of the prostate for benign prostatic hyperplasia: a systematic review with meta-analysis from 2002 to 2012. Eur Urol. 2012;62(2):315–23.
74. Tombal B, De Visccher L, et al. Assessing the risk of unsuspected prostate cancer in patients with benign prostatic hypertrophy: a 13-year retrospective study of the incidence and natural history of T1a-T1b prostate cancers. BJU Int. 1999;84(9):1015–20.
75. Tyson MD, Lerner LB. Safety of holmium laser enucleation of the prostate in anticoagulated patients. J Endourol. 2009;23(8):1343–6.
76. van Rij S, Gilling PJ. In 2013, holmium laser enucleation of the prostate (HoLEP) may be the new 'gold standard'. Curr Urol Rep. 2012;13(6):427–32.
77. Westenberg A, Gilling P, et al. Holmium laser resection of the prostate versus transurethral resection of the prostate: results of a randomized trial with 4-year minimum long-term follow-up. J Urol. 2004;172(2):616–9.
78. Wilson LC, Gilling PJ. From coagulation to enucleation: the use of lasers in surgery for benign prostatic hyperplasia. Nat Clin Pract Urol. 2005;2(9):443–8.
79. Woo HH. Photoselective vaporization of the prostate using the 120-W lithium triborate laser in enlarged prostates (>120 cc). BJU Int. 2011;108(6):860–3.
80. Xia SJ, Zhu J, et al. The treatment of benign prostatic hyperplasia by means of transurethral holmium laser enucleation. Zhonghua Nan Ke Xue. 2003;9(4):257–9.
81. Xia SJ, Zhuo J, et al. Thulium laser versus standard transurethral resection of the prostate: a randomized prospective trial. Eur Urol. 2008;53(2):382–9.
82. Zhang F, Shao Q, et al. Thulium laser versus holmium laser transurethral enucleation of the prostate: 18-month follow-up data of a single center. Urology. 2012;79(4):869–74.

Chapter 8
Emerging Treatments in BPH

Roman Sosnowski and Nikesh Thiruchelvam

Abstract Surgical treatment of BPH is well established. TURP is recognized as the gold standard procedure, and variations now exist in the form of differing energy source to complete prostate resection or enucleation. This chapter outlines newer and experimental techniques in the surgical treatment of BPH. This includes laparoscopic and robotic adenomectomy, urethral lift procedures, and intraprostatic injection of alcohol. The techniques and outcomes are described and given the paucity of long-term outcome and the lack of worldwide experience in these techniques, these techniques are considered to be in their infancy.

Keywords Laparoscopic adenomectomy • Robotic adenomectomy • UroLift • Transurethral ethanol ablation

Laparoscopic Adenomectomy

The European Association of Urology guidelines recommend that open surgery should be the treatment of choice when prostate volume is higher than 80 ml [1]. In recent years, laparoscopy has proved that it could be used for most surgeries in the urological domain, among others in the treatment of BPH [2]. If due to the size of the prostate TURP is not recommended (as prolonged resection can lead to TURP syndrome) or if BPH is accompanied by bladder diverticula or bladder stones or if

R. Sosnowski (✉)
Department of Urology, M. Sklodowska-Curie Memorial Cancer Center,
and Institute of Oncology, Roentgena 5, Warsaw 02-781, Poland
e-mail: roman.sosnowski@gmail.com

N. Thiruchelvam
Department of Urology, Addenbrookes Hospital, Cambridge University
Hospitals NHS Trust, Hills Road, Cambridge, CB2 OQQ, UK
e-mail: nikesh.thiruchelvam@addenbrookes.nhs.uk

it is difficult to insert the resectoscope because of a urethral stricture, laparoscopic adenomectomy may be one of therapeutic options.

In 2002, Mariano et al. presented the first laparoscopic prostatectomy for BPH [3]. In his own technique, he described a transperitoneal route using 5 trocars. The prostate capsule was incised lengthwise, along with the neck of the bladder. The mean operative time was 138 min, mean blood loss was estimated at 330 ml, and the mean amount of the tissue removed during surgery was 131 g. There was a marked improvement in I-PSS and Q_{max}. In 2004, van Velthoven et al. published their experience with laparoscopic adenomectomy, using in 18 patients a slightly different surgical technique which imitated the Millin's method with an average operative time of 145 min, blood loss 192 ml, and mean weight of adenoma resected 47 g [4]. In 2005, Sotelo et al. described 17 cases of laparoscopic simple retropubic prostatectomy [5], while Rey et al. presented ten cases, including three cases which underwent finger-assisted enucleation [6]. After these initial reports, laparoscopic simple prostatectomy has spread.

The Surgical Technique

The laparoscopic approach can be either extra- or intraperitoneal, following a transcapsular or transvesical route. Finger support may be applied for a faster enucleation of large adenomas [7]. The preparation of the patient for the procedure is similar to other laparoscopic urological procedures. Usually, the patient lies on the table in the supine position with the lower limbs in a 30° abduction and in the slight Trendelenburg position. Before the operation a catheter is introduced to drain the bladder.

Various techniques are used in laparoscopy to create the preperitoneal space. In one of them, an incision is made under the navel and CO_2 is insufflated in the extraperitoneal space using a Veress needle (at 12 mmHg) [7]. Another method consists in making a 2 cm upright-midline incision above the pubic arch and using an index finger to navigate a 700 ml self-dilating balloon that dissects the preperitoneal and Retzius space [8]. Next, there is a method that creates the preperitoneal space when after an insertion of a balloon dissector, the retroperitoneal space is brusquely dissected with an introduction of nearly 800–1,200 ml of sterile saline into the balloon. The Hasson trocar is inserted under the umbilicus. The operation can also begin with a primary introduction of the 10 mm infraumbilical port and a laparoscope. A dissection of the preperitoneal space is then completed with the aid of a laparoscope and insufflation. Usually, 4 trocars are introduced (5 or 12 mm) in order to insert a needle for suturing; they are entered in a fan shape (as for extraperitoneal radical prostatectomy). Normally, one 10-mm port is placed infraumbilically as a camera port. Pneumoextraperitoneum is created usually at 12 mmHg. The anterior wall of the prostate and the pelvic fascia are exposed [2]. Next, the dorsal vein complex may be coagulated using bipolar forceps cranially and distantly from the puboprostatic region; alternatively, two hemostatic sutures can be put on these vessels [8].

Using a bladder catheter or a special metal guide introduced into the urethra as a reference point, a limit between the bladder neck and the prostate base is identified. If needed, two hemostatic sutures could be laid on the lateral surface of the prostatic gland at the level of the vesicoprostatic vessels bilaterally. The prostatic capsule is opened 3–4 cm transversally depending on the prostate size, far away from the puboprostatic ligaments (to avoid bleeding from the dorsal vascular plexus), and 1 cm distally to the bladder neck. Hemostatic seams are laid at the 5 and 7 o'clock positions [6]. The capsular cut proceeds in depth until the milky tissue of adenoma can be noticed. With the use of monopolar scissors and the suction irrigation cannula, the plane between prostatic adenoma and the capsule is developed. After developing the anterior plane, a dissection moves laterally and then posteriorly. Sometimes, if there is a need for an improvement of exposure, an incision could be widened in the form of the inverted letter "T" on the prostatic capsule [9]. For enucleation of the lateral lobes, the urethral mucosa is cut circumferentially at the bladder neck. Using a laparoscopic claw grasper, the lateral lobes are grasped. With the aid of the Harmonic scalpel, the surgical avascular capsular plane is developed distally in the direction of the apex, laterally to the posterior plane, and cranially to the bladder neck in the same fashion as during an open procedure in the avascular plane. One of the surgical modifications is the application of two lateral stay seams between the cut prostatic capsule and the Cooper ligament, which then gives a superior image of the fossa and the cleavage plane [10].

When patients present with bladder stones, they can be removed during an intervention through the capsular incision. In cases of significant bladder diverticulum, they could be removed laparoscopically at the same operative session before adenomectomy with no variation in the number or positioning of the operative ports. After an excision of adenoma, one or two corresponding specimens are placed outside the capsule in the lateral prostatic fossas, for example, in the area of the obturator fossa waiting for further removal. Hemostasis is controlled using bipolar or monopolar electrocoagulation for minor vessels and stitches for transcapsular arteries. The prostate fossa is inspected for any remaining nodules of adenoma.

In order to facilitate reepithelialization of the prostatic fossa and for a better control of hemostasis, trigonization of the prostatic fossa is performed using 2–4 stitches laid between the sacral lip of the bladder neck and the posterior surgical capsule. Trigonization eases reepithelialization of the prostate cavity and may also promote hemostasis; nevertheless, it is a challenging surgical step and not always essential [7]. The bladder catheter is then exchanged usually by irrigation or the classic Foley catheter, next the prostatic capsula is remodeled with a running or interrupted suture. Then, a bag sac is introduced by the lateral 10 mm port and the fragmented adenoma placed inside. If adenoma is too big to be entirely removed before extraction, morcellation of the adenoma maybe performed. A drain is placed via a port, and a bag with the specimen is removed after having enlarged the infraumbilical incision to allow for an intact retrieval. A catheter is left inside for up to 5 days as usually in open surgery.

Alternatively, the prostatic capsule can be opened by a longitudinal incision on the anterior aspect of the bladder and prolonged to the anterior surface of the prostatic capsule using scissors, bipolar diathermy, or a harmonic scalpel [10]. Stay sutures are laid between the margins of the open bladder and Cooper's ligament on each side. The adenoma is enucleated, retrigonization of the bladder neck mucosa is performed, and the prostatic capsule and bladder are closed using a running suture [11].

The extraperitoneal transvesical approach is another option on reaching the adenoma. In this procedure, a transverse cystotomy incision is made proximally to the junction of the bladder and prostate. Then, a circular incision is made on the vesical mucosa overlying the prostate lobes, which is deepened until prostate adenoma is identified. Next, adenoma is dissected beneath the capsule. At the end of the procedure, the transverse cystotomy is closed in a watertight manner.

In some cases, particularly of large adenomas or when an operator is at the beginning of the learning curve or there is no clear layer for preparation, instead of using laparoscopic scissors or the Maryland forceps, a finger-assisted technique can be used for dissection of adenoma. After desufflation and the removal of all tools and the camera from the operating field, an index finger is introduced through the suprapubic trocar into the cleavage plane between prostatic adenoma and the capsule. Adenoma is then extirpated using the fingers by blunt dissection analogously to the standard open operation [8, 12, 13]. At this stage of the procedure, raising the prostatic gland by an assistant's finger placed in the rectum helps by directing the prostate to the front and providing counter pressure. An insufficient reach of the finger may be a problem especially in obese patients. The specimen is removed through this incision. Insufflation is started again after the suprapubic incision is closed [14, 15].

Results of Laparoscopic Adenomectomy

The main advantages of laparoscopic adenomectomy are a better control of bleeding due to the magnified view and gas pressure, as well as lower morbidity and less intensive pain compared to open procedure as incisions are smaller and no retractor is used [7]. This results in a better cosmetic effect, smaller risk of wound infections, lower usage of analgesics, consequently shorter hospitalization, and earlier return to normal activities.

Intraoperative complications are rare; the most common include intraoperative bleeding usually of no clinical significance, which occurs in only a few percent of the operated patients with very rare indication for transfusion. Blood loss during the surgery is usually not associated with the amount of enucleated tissue. The tiny blood loss is a consequence of the fact that the gas pressure closes the venous system. This makes performing the hemostatic maneuvers easier before enucleating adenoma. Under these circumstances, more precise dissection and coagulation of the adenomatous cleavage plane is possible [10]. Moreover, a more effective hemostasis should be accomplished due to the magnification from laparoscopy. In total, the standard early complication rate is 14 %, especially when taking into account that most complications were low grade (<II grade in accordance with the Clavien system) [4, 16].

Also, the long-term complications are rare (2.5 % during a 12-month observation, <5 % during a mean 30-month observation) and mainly concern new onset obstructive urinary symptoms, e.g., short presphincteric urethral stenosis, which usually is treated with endoscopic urethrotomy, as well as urinary tract infections such as pyelonephritis, prostatitis, or epididymitis successfully treated conservatively [16].

The functional assessment of the laparoscopic adenomectomy results confirmed that this type of adenomectomy is highly effective for treating the large prostates. Most authors observe a significant increase in Q_{max} compared to the preoperative values rise (the mean increase in Q_{max} by 14.4 – involves the studies presented in Table 8.1) and a dramatic decrease in I-PSS after surgery (the mean decrease in I-PSS by 17.2 – involves the studies presented in Table 8.2). The values of I-PSS remained at the achieved levels during the months following the surgery (3, 6, 12, and longer than 12 months). A similar trend in I-PSS QoL has been observed. The results of the EPIC questionnaire question 32 that has been designed to evaluate patient's satisfaction provided further support for this trend. Patients declared great satisfaction with this intervention starting from the first check-up with no considerable differences during the entire follow-up period [16]. Laparoscopic adenomectomy does not have a significant impact on the change of patient's erectile function assessed among others using IIEF-5 [8]. The persisting consequence of the procedure is retrograde ejaculation; however, this does not have a notable influence on the sexual functions. A change of the PSA concentration was significant between the preoperative and postoperative period, but further observation brought no shifts in the PSA level [16]. A learning curve estimated at about 5–10 procedures is relatively short compared to radical laparoscopic prostatectomy [6]. If conversion is necessary, when the procedure is preperitoneal, there is no need for preparing a new access as the operation is continued in the same space. As laparoscopic skills improve and a number of performed operations increases, the operation time significantly shortens [17].

Comparative studies evaluating laparoscopic adenomectomy and open surgery demonstrate that both treatments are equivalent with regard to the functional results and that laparoscopy provides benefits in the perioperative period such as smaller bleeding, sporadic transfusions, shorter irrigation and catheter permanence times, short hospitalization, few analgesic demands, short convalescence, and a better cosmetic effect [2, 10, 11, 17].

Robotic-Assisted Simple Prostatectomy (RASP)

The first procedures of robotic-assisted simple prostatectomy (RASP) were performed in 2008 [18]. This transvesical technique, described by Sotelo et al. was performed on seven patients with a mean prostatic volume of 77.66 ml (Fig. 8.1a).

Table 8.1 Laparoscopic adenomectomy, data from published series with more than 30 patients

Reference	Study type	No. of patient	Mean follow-up, mounts	Intraoperative transfusion rate, %	Mean operative time, minutes	Mean catheterization time, days	Blood loss, ml	Preoperative prostate volume	Q_{max} change (pre- and postoperative)	I-PSS change (pre- and postoperative)
Mariano et al. [10]	Prospective	60	6	0	138.5	4.6	330	144.5	4.78 – 19.93	28.3 – 5.15
Hoepffner et al. [12]	Retrospective	100	14.05	0	66.34	3.17	250	97.1	6.03 – 26.35	UR – UR
Zhou et al. [8]	Retrospective	45	6	6.6	105	4.6	360.1	85.4	6.1 – 18.7	25.5 – 2.4
Castillo et al. [37]	Prospective	59	30	14.8	123	4.2	415	108.5	UR – UR	18 – 2
Porpiglia et al. [16]	Prospective	78	30	2	103	3.5	333	77	9.8 – 22.7	18.1 – 8.1

UR unreported

8 Emerging Treatments in BPH

Table 8.2 Comparative series between open and laparoscopy adenomectomy from published series

Reference	Study type	Comparative series	No. of patient	Mean follow-up, mounts	Intraoperative transfusion rate, %	Mean operative time, minutes	Mean catheterization time, days	Blood loss, ml	Preoperative prostate volume	Q_{max} change (pre- and postoperative)	I-PSS change (pre- and postoperative)
Porpiglia et al. [2]	Prospective	Open	O – 20	9	O – 20	O – 95.5	O – 5.6	O – 687	O – 115.6	O – 7.7 – 25.4	O – 17.8 – 6.7
			L – 20		L – 20	L – 107.2	L – 6.3	L – 411	L – 94.2	L – 8.8 – 27.2	L – 20.9 – 10.0
Baumert et al. [11]	Retrospective	Open	O – 30	3	3.33	O – 54	O – 6.8	O – 643	O – 106.2	O – UR	O – UR
			L – 30			L – 115	L – 4	L – 367	L – 121.8	L – 8.1 – 24.6	L – 22.4 – 5.7
Garcia-Segui and Gascon Mir [9]	Retrospective	Open	O – 18	1	O – 22	O – 101	O – 7.5	O – 493	O – 114	O – 5.9 – 24.4	O – 24.7 – 6.8
			L – 17		L – 0	L – 135	L – 5.5	L – 250	L – 95	L – 9.3 – 19.7	L – 25.8 – 6.3
McCullough et al. [17]	Prospective	Open	O – 184	UR	O – 10.2	O – 54.7	O – 6.4	O – 400	O – 117	O – UR	O – UR
			L – 96		L – 15.8	L – 95.1	L – 5.2	L – 350	L – 111	L – UR	L – UR
Barret et al. [38][a]	Prospective	Open	O – 60	UR	O – 15	O – 64	O – 6.8	O – 564	O >110	O – UR	O – UR
			L – 60		L – 13	L – 113	L – 4.9	L – 595	L >110	L – UR	L – UR
Peltier et al. [39][a]	Prospective	Open	O – 51	UR	O – UR	O – 90	O – 4	O – 500	O – UR	O – UR – 17.8	O – UR-6
			L – 51		L – UR	L – 149	L – 2	L – 100	L – UR	L – UR – 22	L – UR-3

O open adenomectomy, *L* laparoscopy adenomectomy, *UR* unreported
[a]Only abstract

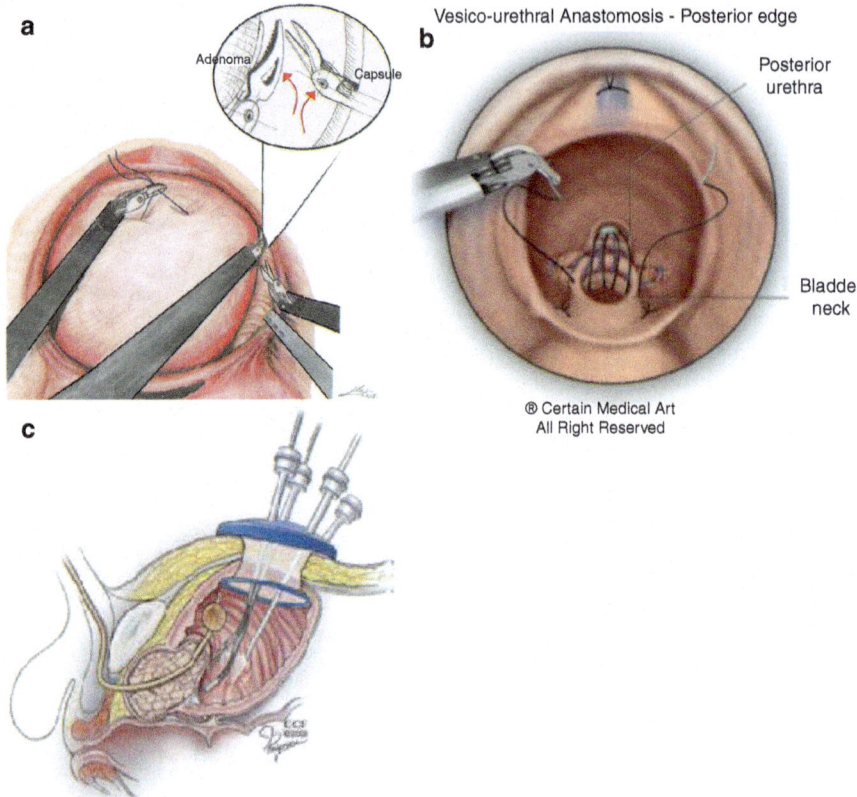

Fig. 8.1 Laparoscopic and robotic adenomectomy. (**a**) Dissection of adenoma in the subcapsular plane (*Source*: Sotelo et al. [18]). (**b**) Modified vesicourethral anastomosis (*Source*: Coelho et al. [20]). (**c**) Robotic adenomectomy using R-Step GelPort inserted in the superior aspect of the bladder (*Source*: Fareed et al. [30])

The mean operation time was 205 min and the mean intraoperative blood loss was 298 ml. Very good functional results were achieved – a reduction by 14.5 points in I-PSS and an increase of Q_{max} by 37.75 ml/s. On this basis, the authors concluded that "Robotic simple prostatectomy is a feasible and reproducible procedure for symptomatic BPH." In the same year, Yuh presented robotic-assisted simple prostatectomy (RASP) in three patients operated using the technique that was similar to the classic Millin's operations; the prostate volume was from 97 to over 600 ml [19]. The mean operation time was 211 min and the intraoperative blood loss was 558 (150–1,125) ml, there were no acute intraoperative or perioperative complications; however, ultimately the patient required a larger extraction incision.

The Surgical Technique

The surgical access and placing of ports in robotic-assisted simple prostatectomy (RASP) is the same as in robotic radical prostatectomy. The operation is performed by applying a transperitoneal six-port technique [20].

Once the retropubic space of Retzius is dissected, the endopelvic fascia is opened laterally to the reflection of the puboprostatic ligaments bilaterally. The dorsal venous complex is ligated. The operation uses the transvesical or prevesical access to adenoma [19, 21–23].

In the prevesical access, the front of the bladder neck is cut proximally to the vesicoprostatic junction. A horizontal incision is made on the vesical mucosa overlying the prostatic lobes at the level of the posterior bladder neck. Then, the plane between adenoma and the prostatic capsule is identified and dissected. Next, the prostatic urethra is transected gently to avoid an injury to the external sphincter and adenoma is removed. Re-trigonization is performed by suturing the posterior edge of the bladder neck mucosa to the posterior edge of the urethra. The classic Foley or the irrigation catheter is introduced during the formation of anastomosis and the prostatic capsule is then closed. The specimen is removed via the primary camera trocar incision [20, 23].

During the transvesical approach, a horizontal cystotomy incision is made proximal to the junction of the bladder and prostate. A horizontal incision is made on the vesical mucosa overlying the prostate lobes. Then, the adenoma is released from the prostatic capsule by cutting apart in the subcapsular plane outer to prostatic adenoma using a combined technique of electrocautery and blunt dissection. After removing the adenoma, the horizontal cystotomy incision is closed in a watertight manner [18].

Modifications of the technique include plication of the posterior prostatic capsule along with modified van Velthoven continuous vesicourethral anastomosis as well as suturing of the front prostatic capsule to the anterior bladder layer [20] (Fig. 8.1b). Another modification is based on the *finger-assisted technique* using open finger enucleation over a 5-cm suprapubic incision.

The Results of Robotic-Assisted Simple Prostatectomy (RASP)

Open adenomectomy performed using the technique of retropubic transvesical or suprapubic transcapsular operation is a recognized treatment of adenomas measuring over 80 ml; however, the procedure is invasive and adenomectomy is carried out by blunt dissection from the capsule, especially in the apical and sphincteric area.

The results of laparoscopic adenomectomy that has been performed since 2002 have improved compared to the open operation in terms of shortening the procedure, reducing the quantity of administered painkillers (analgesia), and the time of a catheter maintenance [6]. However, some restrictions in the laparoscopic technique such as two-dimensional imaging, with merely three degrees of freedom for an instrument maneuver, prolonged standing, and inconvenient operating position contribute to long learning curves and subsequently, slow refinement of laparoscopic skills [24]. Adenomectomy performed using the robotic system – robotic-assisted simple prostatectomy (RASP) – with its advantages such as three-dimensional vision, the Endowrist technology, and the more ergonomic position during the operation, makes both the performance and learning the procedure easier.

Patients subjected to robotic-assisted simple prostatectomy (RASP) had significant improvements in the urinary flow – the mean increase of Q_{max} by 18.6 – involves the studies presented in Table 8.1 and a decrease in I-PSS after surgery (the mean reduction of I-PSS by 15.2 – involves the studies presented in Table 8.1). The duration of the procedure and blood loss are comparable to laparoscopic adenomectomy and in most cases, no blood transfusion was necessary [22] (Table 8.3). By using the *finger-assisted technique*, it is possible to reduce the operative time to 140 min and the blood loss to 250 ml [21]. Hospitalization is short and in most cases the patient is discharged on the first day after the procedure. The patient returns to work very fast, after 13 days on average. Good results of the functional tests are possible to obtain using robotic-assisted simple prostatectomy (RASP) both for small (80 g or less) and bigger (>100 g) prostates [22]. Due to the limited observation time in the presented series (Table 8.3), it is difficult to determine the long-term complications. During a long-term observation, bladder neck stricture can be observed in a small percentage (7.6 %), which can be successfully treated by a transurethral incision [21].

Robotic-assisted simple prostatectomy (RASP) has unquestionable advantages such as minimally invasive approaches, short hospitalization, tiny scar, quick convalescence, and fast return to work. Taking advantage of the benefits brought by robotic surgery, including 6 degrees of freedom, dexterity enhancement, stereovision, and tremor filtering, contributes to more precise and easier operating as well as faster learning of the surgical technique.

Single-Site Surgery

As one of the latest minimally invasive techniques, laparo-endoscopic single-site (LESS) surgery has recently also been used in adenomectomy [25]. The first reports concerned the use of traditional laparoscopic instruments. In 2008, Desai et al. presented the first accounts on single-port transvesical enucleation of the prostate (STEP) carried out by a solitary suprapubic incision using a single-port device (r-Port®) introduced straight into the bladder in three patients having the BPH symptoms [26]. The mean weight of the prostate was 124 g and the operation time was from 6 to 1.5 h with a blood loss from 900 to 250 ml. In the next year, Sotelo et al. performed single-port transvesical enucleation of the prostate (STEP) using r-Port® through the transvesical access forming the working intraperitoneal space [27]. The operation time was 120 min with a blood loss of 200 ml

Table 8.3 Robotic-assisted simple prostatectomy (RASP), data from published series

Reference	Study type	No. of patient	Mean follow-up, mounts	Intraoperative transfusion rate, %	Mean operative time, minutes	Mean catheterization time, days	Blood loss, ml	Preoperative prostate volume	Q_{max} change (pre- and postoperative)	I-PSS change (pre- and postoperative)
Satelo et al. [18]		7	1	14.2	205	7	298	77.66	17.7 – 55.5	22 – 7.5
Yuh et al. [19]	Retrospective	3	UR	0	211	UR	558	323 (one case >600)	UR – UR	14.3 – UR
John et al. [21]		13	13	0	210 (140 with finger-assisted enucleation)	6	500		UR – 23	UR – UR
Uffort and Jensen [40]	Retrospective	15	3	0	128.8	4.6	139.3	46.4	UR – UR	23.79 – 8.13
Matei et al. [41]		15	4.6	O	180	7	50	97.9	7.95 – 25	UR – UR
Sutherland et al. [23]	Retrospective	9	9.25	O	183	13	206	136.5	UR – UR	17.88 – 7.77
Vora et al. [22]		13	7.25	0	179	8.8	219	163.3	4.3 – 19.1	18.1 – 5.3
Coelho et al. [20]	Prospective	6	2	0	90	4.8	208	157	7.75 – 19	19.8 – 5.5
Matei et al. [24]		35	UR	0	180	7	100	96.2	7.5 – 18.3	24 – 5

giving a satisfactory functional result (Q_{max} 85 ml/s). In 2010, Desai et al. described their experiences from the STEP surgery carried out in 34 patients [28]. They obtained good functional results (an increase of Q_{max} from 7.8 to 44 ml/s and a decrease in the I-PSS score from 19 to 3 points). However, the treatments were associated with an intraoperative blood loss, 460 ml on average, along with a need for intraoperative blood transfusion in 15 %. Open conversion was necessary in two patients due to complications, while extension of the skin incision by 1–2 cm had to be done in two of them to expedite apical digital enucleation. The authors demonstrated that STEP is technically feasible but still challenging.

In order to avoid the main limitation of STEP – robotic arm collisions and a small operating space – the set of single-site instruments is applied, which has been designed to be used with the da Vinci® SiSurgical System ed. GelPort® or the intuitive surgical single-port instrument®. Thanks to these solutions collisions are reduced externally as the curved cannula angle the robotic arms aside from each other [29].

Recently, Fareed et al. demonstrated the perioperative and short-term outcomes in nine patients who have been subjected to robotic single-port transvesical enucleation of the prostate (R-STEP) using the da Vinci® S operating system [30]. A 3 cm lower midline incision was made, cystotomy created, and the GelPort positioned in the bladder (Fig. 8.1c). There was a significant postoperative improvement in the flow rates. However, a high-grade (Clavien III–IV) complication was observed in three patients (37.5 %). The authors concluded that despite providing an adequate relief to the bladder outlet obstruction, the procedure carries a high risk of complications and its role still has to be determined.

More recently, a combined approach featuring bipolar enucleation and LESS surgery was applied in the prostate surgery. Rao et al. treated five patients [31]. He used a transurethral bipolar resectoscope as an aid to detach the apical part of the prostate, which facilitated transvesical enucleation. The mean weight of the prostate was 114 g and the operative time is shortened with an increasing experience of an operator and ranged from 45 to 180 min.

Urethral Lift

This technique involves pulling the lateral lobes of the prostate laterally towards the capsule to increase the size of the urethral lumen and overcome the obstruction caused by the enlarged prostatic lobes. Its advantage is that this technique causes immediate relief of obstruction with minimal morbidity.

The technique involves standard cystoscopy. A custom implant delivery device (the UroLift System®) is inserted into the sheath and used to endoscopically compress a lateral prostatic lobe in an anterolateral direction using a non-absorbable monofilament suture with a nitinol capsular tab. The suture-based implant is then delivered and further implants are then placed as required to achieve a visually open urethral lumen. The length of suture is estimated from preoperative transrectal ultrasound of the prostate to ensure the needle enters the prostate capsule. A visual increase in urethral lumen can be seen at the end of the procedure (Fig. 8.2). Patients

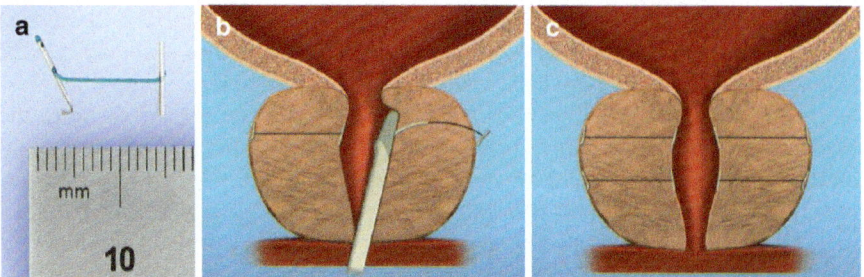

Fig. 8.2 UroLift. (**a**) UroLift implant (non-absorbable monofilament suture with a nitinol capsular tab). (**b**) Implant delivery device inserting implants. (**c**) Final diagrammatic view after placement of 4 implants. The UroLift® System and delivery sequence (Images copyright NeoTract, Inc, with permission)

may or may not be catheterized postoperatively. Key feature of this technique is that it may be performed with local anesthetic and oral sedation [32, 33] and that the urethral end invaginates into the prostate tissue to avoid encrustation.

Early common complications include hematuria, dysuria, and irritative urinary symptoms. Retrograde ejaculation is rare. Later complications uncommonly include UTI and prostatitis and transient erectile dysfunction. Some patients flowing UroLift have undergone TURP with no changes to standard operating technique. Histology around the implants has shown benign changes only.

Short-term efficacy is impressive with around 40 % reduction in I-PSS, 40–50 % improvement in QoL scores and 30 % improvement in peak flow rates. This improvement occurs at 2 weeks and appears to be sustained at 2 years. Although rapid sustained improvement with minimal morbidity and no impotence or incontinence is observed, current unknowns include efficacy in larger prostates (greater than 100 g), long-term follow-up, and any evident changes to prostate histology with long-term implantation. Some of this may be answered by the LIFT study which has to date completed enrolment and is currently in the follow-up phase.

TEAP, Transurethral Ethanol Ablation of the Prostate

Prostatic injection therapy was initially investigated using the transperineal route in the 1960s, but following radiological evidence of extraprostatic extravasation and perineal pain, this route was largely abandoned. There has been recent further interest in this route but this approach has largely been superseded by the transurethral approach. After trying various sclerosants, anhydrous alcohol appears to produce a reproducible host-mediated inflammatory response and localized coagulative necrosis. In addition, it may cause lysis of intraprostatic nerve cells and nerve endings. Improvement in LUTs is observed from the reduction in prostate volume and possibly due to a reduction in intraprostatic alpha-receptors.

Currently, dehydrated alcohol is injected using the ProstaJect® device which is (based on a modified prostate radiofrequency ablation needle) a hollow retractable 22G curved needle which allows for injection of the sclerosant into the prostate using a cystoscope. Injections are placed approximately 1 cm distal to the bladder neck and sometimes a further 2 cm distal to the bladder neck depending on the prostate length. Approximately, an equivalent of 20 % of the prostate volume (as measured by TRUS) is injected. The procedure can be performed under a local anesthetic. Postoperatively, one in five to one in four developed temporary irritative voiding symptoms, retention, or hematuria. Rare adverse events include hemospermia, erectile dysfunction, anejaculation, acute epididymitis, prostatitis, and urethral stricture disease. Of considerable concern is that almost one in ten need a TURP because of lack of improvement of symptoms. Also alarmingly, two significant adverse events have occurred. One patient post TEAP and then TURP has undergone urinary diversion because of bladder necrosis and subsequent urinary leak [34]. Another patient has undergone ureteric reimplantation for distal ureteric stricture following TEAP and then TURP. Despite these events, some reports list no adverse events and encouraging improvements. Maximal results occur at 3 months and appear to be maintained at 12 months. Q_{max} increases from 8.50 to 12 ml/s at 12 months and I-PSS scores improved from 21 to 12. PV can be reduced by up to 16 % at 1 year. Long-term follow-up at 4 years also appears to show ongoing efficacy [35, 36]. The procedure appears to be efficacious in those with LUTs and also those in AUR. Clearly, patients need to be warned that if treatment fails, surgical resection (TURP) is possible but carries a low risk of significant morbidity.

References

1. Oelke M, Bachmann A, Descazeaud A, Emberton M, Gravas S, Michel MC, et al. Guidelines on the management of male lower urinary tract symptoms (LUTS), incl. benign prostatic obstruction (BPO): European Association of Urology. 2012; 40–70. ISBN 978-90-79754-71-7
2. Porpiglia F, Terrone C, Renard J, Grande S, Musso F, Cossu M, et al. Transcapsular adenomectomy(Millin): a comparative study, extraperitoneal laparoscopy versus open surgery. Eur Urol. 2006;49(1):120–6. PubMed PMID: 16310927.
3. Mariano MB, Graziottin TM, Tefilli MV. Laparoscopic prostatectomy with vascular control for benign prostatic hyperplasia. J Urol. 2002;167(6):2528–9. PubMed PMID: 11992078.
4. van Velthoven R, Peltier A, Laguna MP, Piechaud T. Laparoscopic extraperitoneal adenomectomy (Millin): pilot study on feasibility. Eur Urol. 2004;45(1):103–9; discussion 9. PubMed PMID: 14667525.
5. Sotelo R, Spaliviero M, Garcia-Segui A, Hasan W, Novoa J, Desai MM, et al. Laparoscopic retropubic simple prostatectomy. J Urol. 2005;173(3):757–60. PubMed PMID: 15711263.
6. Rey D, Ducarme G, Hoepffner JL, Staerman F. Laparoscopic adenectomy: a novel technique for managing benign prostatic hyperplasia. BJU Int. 2005;95(4):676–8. PubMed PMID: 15705103.
7. Asimakopoulos AD, Mugnier C, Hoepffner JL, Lopez L, Rey D, Gaston R, et al. Laparoscopic treatment of benign prostatic hyperplasia (BPH): overview of the current techniques. BJU Int. 2011;107(7):1168–82. PubMed PMID: 21438981.

8. Zhou LY, Xiao J, Chen H, Zhu YP, Sun YW, Xuan Q. Extraperitoneal laparoscopic adenomectomy for benign prostatic hyperplasia. World J Urol. 2009;27(3):385–7. PubMed PMID: 19082604.
9. Garcia Segui A, Gascon Mir M. Comparative study between laparoscopic extraperitoneal and open adenomectomy. Actas Urol Esp. 2012;36(2):110–6. PubMed PMID: WOS:000300133900009. Spanish.
10. Mariano MB, Tefilli MV, Graziottin TM, Morales CM, Goldraich IH. Laparoscopic prostatectomy for benign prostatic hyperplasia – a six-year experience. Eur Urol. 2006;49(1):127–31; discussion 31–2. PubMed PMID: 16314034.
11. Baumert H, Ballaro A, Dugardin F, Kaisary AV. Laparoscopic versus open simple prostatectomy: a comparative study. J Urol. 2006;175(5):1691–4. PubMed PMID: 16600732.
12. Hoepffner JL, Gaston R, Piechaud T, Rey D. Finger assisted laparoscopic retropubic prostatectomy (Millin). Eur Urol Supp. 2006;5:962–7.
13. Chlosta PL, Varkarakis IM, Drewa T, Dobruch J, Jaskulski J, Antoniewicz AA, et al. Extraperitoneal laparoscopic Millin prostatectomy using finger enucleation. J Urol. 2011;186(3):873–6. PubMed PMID: WOS:000293688300031. English.
14. Rehman J, Khan SA, Sukkarieh T, Chughtai B, Waltzer WC. Extraperitoneal laparoscopic prostatectomy (adenomectomy) for obstructing benign prostatic hyperplasia: transvesical and transcapsular (Millin) techniques. J Endourol. 2005;19(4):491–6. PubMed PMID: 15910264.
15. Slojewski M, Golab A, Galeski M, Sikorski A. Adenomektomia laparoskopowa w leczeniu łagodnego rozrostu stercza. Urol Pol. 2008;61(11):48–54.
16. Porpiglia F, Fiori C, Cavallone B, Morra I, Bertolo R, Scarpa RM. Extraperitoneoscopic transcapsular adenomectomy: complications and functional results after at least 1 year of followup. J Urol. 2011;185(5):1668–73. PubMed PMID: WOS:000289279600037. English.
17. McCullough TC, Heldwein FL, Soon SJ, Galiano M, Barret E, Cathelineau X, et al. Laparoscopic versus open simple prostatectomy: an evaluation of morbidity. J Endourol. 2009;23(1):129–33. PubMed PMID: 19119803.
18. Sotelo R, Clavijo R, Carmona O, Garcia A, Banda E, Miranda M, et al. Robotic simple prostatectomy. J Urol. 2008;179(2):513–5. PubMed PMID: 18076926.
19. Yuh B, Laungani R, Perlmutter A, Eun D, Peabody JO, Mohler JL, et al. Robot-assisted Millin's retropubic prostatectomy: case series. Can J Urol. 2008;15(3):4101–5.
20. Coelho RF, Chauhan S, Sivaraman A, Palmer KJ, Orvieto MA, Rocco B, et al. Modified technique of robotic-assisted simple prostatectomy: advantages of a vesico-urethral anastomosis. BJU Int. 2012;109(3):426–33. PubMed PMID: 21851543.
21. John H, Bucher C, Engel N, Fischer B, Fehr JL. Preperitoneal robotic prostate adenomectomy. Urology. 2009;73(4):811–5. PubMed PMID: 19195694.
22. Vora A, Mittal S, Hwang J, Bandi G. Robot-assisted simple prostatectomy: multi-institutional outcomes for glands larger than 100 grams. J Endourol. 2012;26(5):499–502.
23. Sutherland DE, Perez DS, Weeks DC. Robot-assisted simple prostatectomy for severe benign prostatic hyperplasia. J Endourol. 2011;25(4):641–4. PubMed PMID: 21413877.
24. Matei DV, Brescia A, Mazzoleni F, Spinelli M, Musi G, Melegari S, et al. Robot-assisted simple prostatectomy (RASP): does it make sense? BJU Int. 2012;110(11):E972–9.
25. Autorino R, Kaouk JH, Stolzenburg JU, Gill IS, Mottrie A, Tewari A, et al. Current status and future directions of robotic single-site surgery: a systematic review. Eur Urol. 2013;63(2):266–80. PubMed PMID: 22940173.
26. Desai MM, Aron M, Canes D, Fareed K, Carmona O, Haber GP, et al. Single-port transvesical simple prostatectomy: initial clinical report. Urology. 2008;72(5):960–5. PubMed PMID: 18835633.
27. Sotelo RJ, Astigueta JC, Desai MM, Canes D, Carmona O, De Andrade RJ, et al. Laparoendoscopic single-site surgery simple prostatectomy: initial report. Urology. 2009;74(3):626–30. PubMed PMID: 19604561.
28. Desai MM, Fareed K, Berger AK, Astigueta JC, Irwin BH, Aron M, et al. Single-port transvesical enucleation of the prostate: a clinical report of 34 cases. BJU Int. 2010;105(9):1296–300. PubMed PMID: 20346053.

29. Autorino R, Sosnowski R, De Sio M, et al. Laparo-endoscopic single-site surgery: recent advances in urology. Cent Eur J Urol. 2012;65(4):204–11.
30. Fareed K, Zaytoun OM, Autorino R, White WM, Crouzet S, Yakoubi R, et al. Robotic single port suprapubic transvesical enucleation of the prostate (R-STEP): initial experience. BJU Int. 2012;110(5):732–7. PubMed PMID: 22340135.
31. Rao P, Desai M, Sotelo R, Rao P, Liu C. Hybrid LESS prostatectomy for BPH: a combined technique. Urology. 2011;78(3):64.
32. Chin PT, Bolton DM, Jack G, Rashid P, Thavaseelan J, Yu RJ, et al. Prostatic urethral lift: two-year results after treatment for lower urinary tract symptoms secondary to benign prostatic hyperplasia. Urology. 2012;79(1):5–11. PubMed PMID: 22202539. Epub 2011/12/29. eng.
33. Barkin J, Giddens J, Incze P, Casey R, Richardson S, Gange S. UroLift system for relief of prostate obstruction under local anesthesia. Can J Urol. 2012;19(2):6217–22. PubMed PMID: 22512970. Epub 2012/04/20. eng.
34. Grise P, Plante M, Palmer J, Martinez-Sagarra J, Hernandez C, Schettini M, et al. Evaluation of the transurethral ethanol ablation of the prostate (TEAP) for symptomatic benign prostatic hyperplasia (BPH): a European multi-center evaluation. Eur Urol. 2004;46(4):496–501; discussion 501–2. PubMed PMID: 15363567. Epub 2004/09/15. eng.
35. Sakr M, Eid A, Shoukry M, Fayed A. Transurethral ethanol injection therapy of benign prostatic hyperplasia: four-year follow-up. Int J Urol. 2009;16(2):196–201. PubMed PMID: 19054163. Epub 2008/12/05. eng.
36. El-Husseiny T, Buchholz N. Transurethral ethanol ablation of the prostate for symptomatic benign prostatic hyperplasia: long-term follow-up. J Endourol. 2011;25(3):477–80. PubMed PMID: 21355774. Epub 2011/03/02. eng.
37. Castillo OA, Bolufer E, López-Fontana G, Sánchez-Salas R, Fonerón A, Vidal-Mora I, et al. Prostatectomía simple (adenomectomía) por vía laparoscópica: experiencia en 59 pacientes consecutivos. Actas Urol Esp. 2011;35(7):434–7.
38. Barret E, Rozet F, Cathelineau X, Vallancien G. The morbidity of laparoscopic versus open simple prostatectomy. J Endourol. 2006;20(2):A271-A. PubMed PMID: WOS:000239906201342. English.
39. Peltier A, Hoffmann P, Hawaux E, Entezari K, Deneft F, van Velthoven R. Laparoscopic extraperitoneal Millin' s adenomectomy versus open retropubicadenomectomy: a prospective comparison. Eur Urol Suppl. 2007;6(2):163.
40. Uffort EE, Jensen JE. Robotic-assisted laparoscopic simple prostatectomy: an alternative minimal invasive approach for prostate adenoma. J Robot Surg. 2010;4:7–10.
41. Matei DV, Spinelli MG, Nordio A, Brescia A, Crisan N, Coman I. Robotic simple prostatectomy. Eur Urol Supp. 2010;9(2):337.

Chapter 9
Managing the Complex/Difficult Cases

Sascha A. Ahyai and Kathrin Simonis

Abstract Although LUTS due to BPH is not often a life-threatening condition, the impact of LUTS/BPH on quality of life can be significant and should not be underestimated. The primary goal in BPH/LUTS treatment in older patients is to alleviate the symptoms, the recreation of quality of life, and to alter disease progression. When selecting an appropriate treatment, age and comorbidities are important factors. Due to an aging population, we have to face complex patients with BPH/LUTS and cardiovascular diseases and anticoagulant therapy with a high perioperative risk, patients with neurogenic LUTS, or patients who have a history of previous BPH surgery.

Keywords BPH • LUTS • Comorbidities • Detrusor failure • Parkinson • TURP

Introduction

LUTS are common in the elderly man. Today, approximately 25 % of all men aged between 40 and 79 years suffer from LUTS, but due to our aging population, it will be around 50 % in 2,025 [1]. In the majority of the elderly men, the age-related growth of the prostate is responsible for LUTS. This was demonstrated in the Olmsted County Study where the presence of moderate-to-severe LUTS was associated with the development of acute urinary retention as a symptom of benign prostatic hyperplasia (BPH) progression, increasing from a prevalence of 6.8 episodes per 1,000 patient-years of follow-up in the overall population to a rate of 34.7 episodes in men aged 70 years or older [2]. Although LUTS is not often

---

S.A. Ahyai • K. Simonis (✉)
Department of Urology, University Medical Center Hamburg,
Martinistraße 52, 20246 Hamburg, Germany
e-mail: sahyai@uke.de; k.simonis@uke.de

a life-threatening condition, the impact of LUTS on quality of life (QoL) can be significant and should not be underestimated [3]. The primary goal in LUTS treatment is to alleviate the symptoms, recreate QoL, and prevent disease progression. Therefore, bothered LUTS patients normally receive mono- or combined medical therapy according to the prostate size and predominance of filling, voiding, and postvoiding symptom. However, medical therapy may also just postpone surgery; as in 50–60 % of all patients undergoing BPH surgery, the main indication is medical treatment failure. Due to medical therapy, but also due to the demographic shift to an aging population in general, we urologists are increasingly confronted with complex patients: Elderly male seeking help for LUTS, having age-related comorbidities such as cardiovascular diseases but also neurogenic disorders and an enlarged prostate, or patients who are symptomatic despite previous BPH surgery. How shall we ideally treat these patients? In such complex patients a detailed diagnostic workup is of major importance, overall as there is increasing evidence that the etiology of LUTS is multifactorial. Approximately 25–50 % of men with histologically proven BPH suffer from LUTS [4], but only 50 % of them are affected by bladder outlet obstruction [5]. LUTS may be due to structural or functional abnormalities in one or more parts of the lower urinary tract but can also result from abnormalities of the peripheral and/or central nervous system. Cardiovascular, respiratory, or renal dysfunction/disease may also cause LUTS. Finally, the classical symptoms of LUTS can be mimicked by other issues such as overactivity or hypocontractility of the detrusor muscle [3].

In this chapter we want to discuss how to proceed ideally with male patients suffering from LUTS on the one hand and having a history of (1) cardiovascular disease and need of anticoagulant therapy, (2) Parkinson's disease (PD), (3) hypocontractile detrusor, or (4) previous prostate surgery on the other hand. We consider these patients to be complex and named this chapter accordingly. It is unnecessary to mention that urodynamics (UD) (cystomanometry and pressure-flow study) in these complex/neurogenic patients are mandatory – to indicate or to rule out surgery, or vice versa – to prevent the risks of unnecessary not indicated therapies, let it be conservative or invasive.

Cardiovascular (CV) Comorbidities

Manifestations of arteriosclerosis are coronary heart disease, peripheral arterial disease, and ischemic strokes. Cardiovascular diseases (CVD) are the most frequent cause of death (25–55 %) worldwide [6]. However, in Europe and North America, its mortality decreased considerably during the last years due to prevention and progress in (acute) therapy. The prevalence of CVD and hypertension is increasing with age as well as LUTS and BPH. And similarly to LUTS and BPH, with the growing life expectancy, the proportion of patients with relevant cardiovascular comorbidities will still increase substantially in the near future. In the Western world life expectancy is increasing due to today's improved and consequent treatment modalities. As a result people can grow older. This implies a higher risk of developing atrial fibrillation, hereditary or acquired thrombophilia, pathology of the myocardium or valves etc and mostly without drastic limitations in quality of life (QoL). As a consequence for us urologists, there is an increasing proportion of patients on anticoagulation therapy and suffering from LUTS at the same time. As the surgical risk in these patients is increased, the primary treatment option in this patient cohort is to alleviate LUTS suggestive for BPH and to prevent disease progression overall acute urinary retention, chronic renal failure, or recurrent urinary tract infection. Regarding medical treatment the altered drug metabolism of elderly and morbid patients as well side effects and interaction with other medication has to be considered. Among the a1-AR antagonists, tamsulosin does not show interactions with several antihypertensive agents and is well tolerated by older patients [7]. In the MTOPS trial the efficacy of the combination therapy of a1-AR antagonist for rapid symptom relief and 5-alpha-reductase inhibitor to prevent disease progression was clearly demonstrated also in the long term. However, treating such patients becomes more challenging when conservative, medical therapy fails; urodynamic pressure-flow studies show significant benign prostatic obstruction (BPO); or surgical therapy is also indicated in high-risk anticoagulated patients for recurrent hematuria, infection, urinary retention, or deterioration of the upper urinary tract. In these patients overall the cardiovascular and bleeding risks must weighed against surgical benefits.

Urethral or suprapubic catheterization is an option for high-risk patients that are ineligible for surgery and suffer from chronic urinary retention. However, long-term catheterization is associated with considerable costs both to the patient and the health service [8]. Therefore, in these patients prostatic stents may be an alternative. The stent placement is usually performed under regional or topical anesthesia – they may be either permanent or temporary. Systematic reviews of epithelializing and thermo-expandable metallic stents demonstrate efficacy and safety. Unfortunately, due to inadequate follow-up (FU) data, durability of this treatment (over 1 year) is still pending [9].

As long-term data is still missing, prostatic stents should still be considered as an investigational procedure when offered to a patient. Other minimally invasive therapies are transurethral microwave therapy (TUMT) and transurethral needle ablation (TUNA). Under the topic effect of heat TUMT leads to a coagulation necrosis of the prostate tissue and denervation of alpha-receptors, reducing BPO and LUTS. Microwave radiation is emitted through an intraurethral antenna. Contraindications are, i.e., a prostate middle lobe, prostate cancer, neurogenic bladder dysfunction, and prostate volume less than 30 ml or more than 100 ml. Endoscopy before TUMT is mandatory to exclude the presence of a prostate middle lobe. Treatment is well tolerated, although most patients report perineal discomfort and urinary urgency. A Cochrane systematic review comparing TURP with TUMT reports that catheterization time, incidence of dysuria/urgency, and urinary retention were significantly less with TURP. The incidence of hospitalization, hematuria, clot retention, transfusions, TUR syndrome, and urethral strictures were significantly less for TUMT [10]. Long-term data featuring the improvement of symptom score and urinary flow rate is still missing [7]. In TUNA low-level radiofrequency energy is delivered via

Procedure	Bleeding	Capsular perforation	Conversion to TURP	Injury of the mucosa	Transfusion	TUR syndrome	Total
TURP, % (range)	0.3 (0–7.7)	0.1 (0–2.7)	0.0	0.0	2.0 (0–9)	0.8 (0–5)	3.2
Bipolar TURP, % (range)	0.0	0.0	0.0	0.0	1.9 (0–3.7)	0.0	1.9
Bipolar TUVP, % (range)	0.0	0.0	0.0	0.0	0.5 (0–2)	0.0	0.5
HoLEP, % (range)	0.0	0.2 (0–2)	0.0	3.3 (0.0–18.2)	0.0	0.0	3.5
KTP, % (range)	0.0	0.0	3.5 (0–8)	0.0	0.0	0.0	3.5

TURP transurethral resection of the prostate, *TUR* transurethral resection, *TUVP* transurethral vaporisation of the prostste, *HoLEP* holmium laser enucleation of the prostate, *KTP* potassium-titanyl-phosphate.

Fig. 9.1 Treatment-specific intraoperative complications of selected surgical LUTS treatment, according to Ahyai et al. [12a]. Modified with permission from Elsevier

needles into the prostate leading to a coagulation necrosis. Recent studies show that TUNA significantly improved IPSS and Qmax referring to baseline values, but in comparison to TURP this improvement was significantly lower at 12 months. TUMT and TUNA are options for older patients with comorbidities such as CVD and anticoagulation who are unfit for a spinal or general anesthesia, since both procedures can be performed under sedoanalgesia and topical anesthesia. However, high-risk LUTS patients who cannot have surgery/spinal or general anesthesia have become rare in modern medicine and so has the availability of TUMT and TUNA.

Surgery for benign prostatic enlargement (BPE) is an elective surgery. Generally, prostatic surgery has a (high) risk of interventional bleeding. Transurethral resection of the prostate (TURP) is considered as the reference standard of treating BPE. However, according to its complication rate, it is contraindicated for patients who are at high surgical and anesthetic risk, in particular for patients on chronic anticoagulants [7]. Despite technological advances the rate of blood transfusions after TURP remains significant at 2–9.5 % depending on prostate size in contemporary series [11]. Looking at a meta-analysis of intraoperative complications comparing TURP and other transurethral minimal invasive therapies (Fig. 9.1) demonstrates that the risk of intraoperative bleeding and transfusion is lower in patients undergoing kalium-titanyl-phosphate (KTP) laser vaporization and holmium laser enucleation of the prostate (HoLEP) [12a]. The exclusion of the transurethral resection syndrome and the improved hemostatic properties of the KTP laser and holmium:YAG lasers, which led to comparatively significantly mean shorter catheter and hospital time, are the main reasons why patients with CVD, who cannot stop anticoagulation before BPH surgery, should undergo KTP laser vaporization, HoLRP (holmium laser resection of the prostate), or HoLEP according to EAU Guidelines [3]. It was Reich et al. in 2005 who initially proposed photoselective KTP laser vaporization of the prostate in 66 high-risk anticoagulated patients [12]. The mean hemoglobin dropped from 13.9 to 13.0 g/dl and no patient needed blood transfusion or reintervention due to bleeding. In fact, five patients died of cardiopulmonary reasons during the mean follow-up of 12 months, which underlined the poor medical condition of this prospective study cohort. Another study, which underlines the use of the GreenLight Laser vaporization in anticoagulated patients with LUTS, was published by Chung et al. [13]. Indication for surgery was in 65 % LUTS refractory to medical therapy, in 27 % urinary retention, in 4 % recurrent hematuria, and in 2 % bladder stones and recurrent urinary tract infection. Mean ASA score was 3 with 19 % of the patients on warfarin, 62 % on acetylsalicylic acid, 12 % on clopidogrel, and 7 % on two or more anticoagulants. Of the 162 patients in total, none needed blood transfusion for an immediate complication, but 2 % after delayed bleeding. One patient needed Willebrand factor and another patient reoperation for bleeding fulguration [13]. The functional results after 1 year of FU were acceptable with a mean International Prostatic Symptom Score (IPSS) of 7.3, maximum urinary flow rate (Qmax) of 15 ml/s, and postvoid residual urine (PVR) of 70 ml. One might argue that the rather moderate improvement of Qmax and PVR was owned to the quite high mean baseline prostate volume (91 g) of the study cohort. In contrast to HoLEP, there is controversy about the safety and efficacy profile when using photoselective vaporization in larger prostates (e.g., 60 g) [14]. Therefore, in an anticoagulated patient with a large prostate, HoLEP might be favored. There is one retrospective analysis suggesting excellent hemostatic properties in these high-risk patients with no blood transfusion and no statistical difference in bleeding complications between the coumadin, aspirin, and control group [15] and one prospective case series with a 10 % transfusion rate suggesting that HoLEP is relatively safe and effective for treating patients on oral anticoagulation or therapeutical subcutaneous low-molecular-weight heparin (LMWH). Taken together, one could summarize that patients with CVD and anticoagulation who need invasive BPH surgery should undergo photoselective vaporization or HoLEP especially when the prostate is large. However, the data is very limited and predominantly based on the results of non-anticoagulated patients. We have different types of anticoagulation therapies (vitamin K antagonists: warfarin/coumadin, heparin; thrombocyte inhibitors – aspirin, clopidogrel, and the just recently introduced new direct oral anticoagulants. Obviously the strategies before elective surgery are different depending on the specific anticoagulant. Most patients on warfarin and coumadin are bridged before surgery with LMWH. Depending on their CVD, the dose of LMWH and its application interval can or need to be modified also according to the surgical risk of bleeding. According to the European Society for Cardiology (ESC), in patients with atrial fibrillation who leave the therapeutical INR to a subtherapeutical INR, LMWH can be paused for 2 days.

However, recommendation concerning indication for anticoagulant therapy and the degree of thromboembolic risk and perioperative risk for discontinuation of oral anticoagulation should be based individually on cardiology consultation. We urologists have to bear in mind that due to anticoagulation therapy, it might be worthwhile to postpone surgery if anticoagulant therapy can be paused or reduced again in the future of the patient.

In summary, medical therapy and increased life expectancy have translated into a LUTS population with more CVD requiring active anticoagulation. In these patients TURP is contraindicated due to increased bleeding risk. Instead extended medical or minimal invasive therapy should be offered to these risk patients after preferably complete UD. In patients with significant BPO or absolute indication for prostate surgery, who are unfit for general anesthesia catheterism, prostatic stents, TUMT, or TUNA might be an option. Those patients who are eligible for anesthesia (interestingly, in clinical trials spinal anesthesia vs. general anesthesia does not show advantages in patients with CVD [16]) should be offered laser prostatectomy.

These recommendations rely predominantly on the good hemostatic properties shown overall for the photoselective KTP laser vaporization and HoLEP. Certainly, patients' characteristics such as age, prostate size, personal preference, and availability of the specific lasers have to be considered. Other laser (thulium and diode laser) might also become alternatives in these specific patients. However, the corroboration of their promising results even in non-anticoagulated patients by comparative randomized trials is still pending.

Neurogenic Comorbidities

Parkinson's Disease

Parkinson's disease (PD) is a neurodegenerative disorder associated with loss of dopaminergic neurons mainly in the substantia nigra, but may also affect other parts of the brain or other neurotransmitters apart from the dopaminergic system. Patients with PD have a high prevalence of LUTS (27–39 %) according to validated questionnaires. The most reported symptoms are nocturia (86 %), urinary frequency (71 %), urinary urgency (68 %), und urge incontinence (more than 40 %) [17]. Since PD and BPE are relatively common disorders in older men, it is clinically difficult to answer to what extent LUTS in a male PD individual are neurogenic and/or non-neurogenic. Therefore, baseline UD is a must before considering therapy. In patients with PD, the most common finding in UD is detrusor overactivity (DO) [18]. In PD the neurodegeneration in the nigrostriatal dopamine system removes the tonic inhibitory control over the pontine micturition center leading to decreased bladder capacity and DO [19]. However, clinically bladder dysfunction in PD occurs predominantly after the appearance of motor disorders. And from recent studies we know, that LUTS in Parkinson's disease are related to the extent of dopamine deficiency [20] and the state of neurological disability [21]. Though less frequent than storage symptoms, also voiding symptoms are more prevalent in PD patients when compared to control group. However, measurements of postvoid residual urine in PD patients are low [22]. Although impaired relaxation of the urethral sphincter has been suggested to result in voiding dysfunction [23], interestingly urodynamic studies show that bladder outlet obstruction is not very common in PD [24] as detrusor activity during voiding is weak and detrusor sphincter dyssynergia (DSD) absent [22]. Therefore, renal damage in patients with PD seems less likely, and regular UD less important than in patients with, e.g., multiple sclerosis.

Pharmacological treatment of Parkinson's disease may affect lower urinary tract function. The reported data from recent studies is controversial [25]. DO improved after administration of apomorphine and to a lesser extent after levodopa [26]. Another study showed that in advanced Parkinson's disease with the on-off phenomenon, DO worsened with levodopa in some patients and improved in others [27]. In advanced Parkinson's disease levodopa impairs DO but also improves bladder emptying by increasing detrusor contractility [28]. Selective anticholinergic drugs in PD are indicated when overactive bladder (OAB) does not respond to levodopa or dopamine receptor agonists. Monitoring PVR and cognitive function is then essential to balance possible side effects and improved quality of life due to reduction of OAB. Also, treatment of nocturia with desmopressin in PD needs close follow-up. In 2011, Giannantoni et al. updated their preliminary findings of intradetrusor injection of botulinum toxin type A in patients with PD [29]. The authors could demonstrate significantly decreased day- and nighttime urinary frequency and number of urinary incontinence episodes and increased QoL in eight patients (one male). Before the intradetrusor injection of botulinum toxin type A, all eight PD patients were refractory to at least two anticholinergic agents. Also objective cystometry showed efficacy up to the 6-month FU. Despite using only 100 IU of botulinum toxin type A, two female patients needed transient catheterism due to increased PVR. Still, these results are promising overall for PD patients who are refractory of or have relevant side effects of anticholinergic first-line therapy.

If voiding symptoms in male patients with Parkinson's disease have failed medical treatment and pressure-flow studies show significant (coincident) BPO, surgical therapy needs to be discussed [25]. In 1988, Staskin et al. reported a de novo urinary incontinence rate of 20 % after TURP in patients with Parkinson's disease. The major risk of incontinence was a lack of voluntary sphincter control [30]. According to the high incontinence rate, TURP was considered as unsuitable for patients with PD.

However, a more recent study, published by Roth et al. in 2006, showed that of 23 PD patients undergoing transurethral resection of the prostate (TURP), none experienced de novo urinary incontinence, and at a median FU of 3 years, TURP was still successful in 70 % of the patients. Therefore, PD should no longer be considered as a contraindication for TURP as long as the neurological diagnosis PD is correct and not mistaken with multiple system atrophy (MSA). The pathogenesis of LUTS is different in both neurodegenerative diseases. MSA leads to a wide degeneration of dopaminergic and nondopaminergic areas involving lower urinary tract function including the intermediolateral cell column (neurons innervating the internal sphincter and the bladder) and the Onuf's nucleus (neurons innervating the external sphincter) [31]. Urethral or anal sphincter electromyography is recommended to support the diagnosis of MSA as a selective atrophy of the anterior horn cells that innervate the urethral and anal sphincter [32]. Looking at the adverse outcome of TURP according to the Staskin data from today's perspective, it seems likely that the TURP patients with de novo incontinence rather had MSA than PD [33], overall as Staskin et al. identified a lack of voluntary sphincter control as the major risk factor of incontinence in their study cohort [30]. As a result in patients with PD and BPO, the surgeon should perform an orientating neurological examination including digital rectal examination to exclude flaccid anal sphincter tonus.

In summary, LUTS are common in patients with PD. PD patients referred from the neurologists due to LUTS refractory to dopamine modulation are candidates for UD. DO is the most common finding in PD and can be treated similar to idiopathic OAB with anticholinergics as first-line therapy or intradetrusor injection with 100 IU of botulinum toxin type A as second-line therapy. If UD after failure of

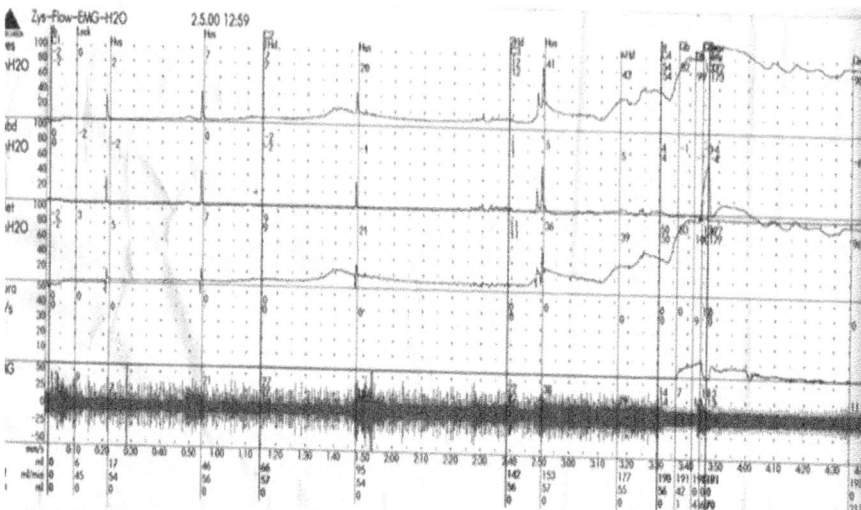

Fig. 9.2 Cystometry and pressure-flow study of a patient with Morbus Parkinson's disease, showing DO and significant detrusor overactivity and outlet obstruction

pharmacological treatment shows BPO, surgical desobstruction can be considered if the diagnosis of PD is secure and voluntary sphincter control is present. Figure 9.2 demonstrates the cystometry and pressure-flow study of a male patient with PD showing DO and significant BPO (Fig. 9.2).

Detrusor Failure

Several recent studies have shown that there is no correlation between LUTS and the presence of obstruction. Uroflowmetry and postvoid residual urine volume are simple tests that can indicate bladder outlet obstruction (BOO) [34]. However, 25–30 % of men with decreased flow are not obstructed [35]. Voiding difficulties can be categorized in impaired detrusor contractility or BOO; both cause a decreased uroflow. Elevated postvoid residual urine (PVR) is more typical for detrusor failure (DF) than for BOO [36]. UD are considered necessary to differentiate between DF and BOO [34]. DF is the inability to empty the bladder sufficiently due to detrusor muscle weakness. Hence, the first clinical sign of DF is urinary retention with increased postvoid residual urine, which finally may lead to acute urinary retention, hydronephrosis, and renal failure in its extreme. Persistent BOO may be the cause of DF by damaging the innervation and smooth muscle. Thus, behind the UD diagnosis of DF – with low pressure and low flow – might also stand a previous long-lasting BOO. Even though UD are the gold standard for bladder outlet obstruction and other voiding and storage abnormalities responsible for LUTS and voiding dysfunction especially in patients with neurogenic disorders [34], UD are not capable to detect BOO in patients with DF and cannot predict individual outcome in such patients when submitted for surgery (e.g., TURP). It is generally known that patients with DF have poorer voiding outcomes after prostatectomy [37], and some advocate that these patients should be arbitrarily excluded from surgery and rather be candidates for lifelong intermittent self-catheterization or suprapubic catheterism. In elderly patients voiding dysfunction is very common. Structural changes in the bladder belong to the aging process. Maximum bladder capacity decreases with age because of decreased concentrations of smooth muscle fibers and other connective tissues in the detrusor. Decreased supra pontine inhibition may result in increased detrusor contractility due to unopposed neural activity. Urinary retention may be caused by decreased afferent activity which leads to decreased detrusor contractility and poor emptying of the bladder [38]. Therefore, Blatt et al. tried to investigate better tools to select patients that benefit from TURP [39]. It is known that in patients with urinary retention due to BOO, there is also an element of myogenic detrusor failure. Previous ultrastructural studies of the detrusor demonstrated consistent changes in the detrusor muscle of patients with voiding dysfunction [40]. True pathological ultrastructural features may be changes to the architecture, interstitium, myocyte, or cell junction of the detrusor muscle. Blatt et al. identified ultrastructural changes in the detrusor of patients with DF and BOO. These changes were correlated with urodynamic findings and clinical outcome: Four ultrastructural features correlated significantly with each other and with voiding outcome following TURP, including muscle cell size, muscle cell shape, abnormal fascicle arrangement, and collagenosis. When all four features were absent, a patient had an 84 % chance of voiding after TURP. According to their findings the authors recommend detrusor muscle biopsy for ultrastructural analysis as a useful tool for selecting patients with DF that will or will not benefit from surgery [39]. However, costs and expertise in detrusor electron microscopy are the limiting drawbacks. More realistic to gain access into clinical practice are ultrasound measurements of the detrusor wall. So far all studies addressing bladder and BOO showed that bladder wall thickening is associated with BOO and that even the increase of detrusor wall thickness (DWT) correlates well with the degree of BOO. Oelke et al. showed that a standardized measurement of the DWT by transabdominal ultrasound is able to predict BOO. Calculation of positive predictive values showed that 94 % of patients with DWT ≥2 mm had BOO [41].

As UD cannot differentiate between patients who have pure DF or DF and BOO, DWT assessment might be a helpful marker. A recent study published by Huang et al. assessed the predictive value of resistive index (RI), DWT, and ultrasound-estimated bladder weight (UEBW) regarding the outcome after TURP in a multivariable model. Predictive accuracy according to ROC analyses was 72 % for UEBW, 76 % for DWT, and 82 % for RI. For clinical practice the authors stated that patients with UEBW <42 g, DWT <15 mm, and RI < 0.64 are at high risk for unfavorable outcome after TURP [42]. The dilemma of these promising noninvasive measurements is that they were used first to predict BOO and secondly to predict surgical outcome, as there is enough evidence that the degree of BOO is the most critical for surgical efficacy. However, it remains unknown how these predictors are influenced by detrusor underactivity or DF. Therefore, they should be assessed prospectively in a multicenter trial in patients with BPE who demonstrate DF at pressure-flow studies. Generally spoken, until there are no reliable investigations to predict outcome of surgical desobstruction in patients with DF, patients need to be informed accordingly. Two recent studies reported that 60 % of the patients with DF were satisfied with the surgical outcome. In detail Ou et al. found significant improvements in symptoms (IPSS, QOL) and urodynamic parameters in patients with preoperatively diagnosed DF after TURP [43]. It might also be a valuable concept to suggest preliminary clean intermittent self-catheterism (CISC) in patients with chronic urinary retention (CUR) and low voiding pressure before surgical therapy. A prospective randomized trial published by Ghalayini et al. emphasized the usefulness of CISC in patients with CUR before TURP ensuring the recovery of bladder function. Interestingly, those patients with persisting low voiding pressure on UD (cutoff <40) after 6 months of CISC had still adverse outcome after surgery [44].

Taken together, patients with a DF are at higher risk for poorer voiding outcomes after TURP than those with preserved detrusor function [39]. To operate on patients with DF is still a matter of debate. In patients with DF UD is not capable to identify patients who might benefit from surgery, since low voiding pressure can be explained by DF or DF and coexisting BOO. New predictors such as DWT might – from a rational point of view – be interesting but need to be investigated in such a specific patients' cohort. So long elderly male patients with DF need to be informed that they might not benefit from prostate surgery and will still need CISC. Therefore, it might be wise to start CISC before considering TURP in patients with DF for a period of 3–6 months, hoping that on repeat UD bladder function has restored. Finally, patients who are likely to have nonobstructive urinary retention/DF before or finally after TURP should be informed about the possibility of sacral neuromodulation therapy as a 70 % successful minimally invasive treatment option to reduce substantially the catheterized PVR volumes and hence the intervals of CISC in the short and long term [45]. The exact mechanism of sacral neuromodulation is not yet completely understood. However, sacral neuromodulation is not without risks even if intraoperative complications are rare. Postoperative complications occur in up to 30 % of patients. The most frequent reported problems are pain, infection, and lead migration [38].

Prior BPH Surgery

According to Emberton et al., up to one third of patients post prostatectomy have unfavorable outcome [46]. The outcome of prostatectomy correlates well with degree of preoperative BOO and is less favorable in patients with equivocal obstruction and detrusor over- and underactivity [47]. Persisting LUTS after prior BPH surgery may be due to DO (24–63 %), residual obstruction (9–36 %), detrusor underactivity/DF (9–55 %), and poor relaxation of the urethra (19 %) [48, 49].

This variety of causes for persisting or de novo LUTS implies the need of UD investigation in these post-prostatectomy patients, overall as treatment differs entirely according to the specific diagnosis found at UD.

In case of persisting BOO, repeat surgery is indicated. Up to now there are only few studies investigating patients with prior BPH surgery. Recurrent prostatic obstruction usually seems to affect elderly patients who might also be on anticoagulant therapy or have associating cardiovascular diseases. This might raise the question if a secondary operation seems to be safe, feasible, and efficient. Secondary surgery in recurrent BPH can be a technical challenge because of disturbed anatomical landmarks [50]. Especially in comorbid patients minimal invasive surgery might be considered. In a recent study, Elshal et al. analyzed patients with history of previous prostate surgery who underwent secondary HoLEP compared to patients with no previous prostate surgery [50]. In all patients with prior BPH surgery, urodynamics and pressure-flow studies were performed. Postoperatively, there was a comparable significant improve of Qmax, IPSS, IQOL, and PVR at all points of follow-up in both groups. Overall there were slightly more postoperative complications (acute urinary retention) in the group with prior surgery. Postoperative stress urinary incontinence was found in 6.5 % of all patients after secondary surgery (vs. 4.5 %). Recurrent obstruction occurred in 5.2 % (vs. 4 %). As shown by this recently publish study, patients undergoing secondary surgery for recurrent BOO should be informed about an increased risk of adverse events such as stress urinary incontinence.

Preoperative DO is a common finding: ranging from 25 % in patients without BOO to 62 % in patients with BOO [51]. Post prostatectomy the incidence decreases to about one fourth according to the data of Abrams et al. [52], whereas 10 % of the patients may demonstrate de novo DO [53]. Persisting or de novo DO hinders symptomatic improvement after surgery.

In general these patients are bothered by idiopathic overactive bladder syndrome (OAB). The likelihood that DO resolves after surgery increases if DO was associated with BOO and decreases with preoperative severity [47]. As OAB correlates with increasing age as well in men as in women, aging seems to be a major reason for DO [54]. This could also explain why patients at long-term FU after previous BPH surgery become symptomatic again, despite no evidence of recurrent BOO. Post-prostatectomy patients with OAB due to DO are generally treated conservatively with antimuscarinics. In patients who are refractory to this treatment, escalation as newly suggested for idiopathic OAB with 100 IU may be indicated [55] or alternatively sacral neuromodulation therapy can be indicated [45]. Patients with LUTS after previous BPH surgery due to DF may finally need CISC after cystoscopic exclusion of residual prostatic tissue or urethral stricture. In case of nonobstructive urinary retention, sacral neuromodulation therapy has a good outcome in these patients as describe above.

In summary, persisting LUTS or unfavorable outcome after previous prostate surgery might be explained by persisting or recurrent BOO but in the majority of cases is explained by DO and DF. Therefore, to prevent unnecessary redo BPH surgery with potential side effects, UD are obligatory in symptomatic patients with previous BPH.

References

1. McNicholas T. Management of symptomatic BPH in the UK: who is treated and how? Eur Urol. 1999;36:33–9.
2. McVary K. BPH: epidemiology and comorbidities. Am J Manag Care. 2006;12(5 Suppl):122.
3. Wei J, Calhoun E, Jacobsen S. Urologic diseases in America project: benign prostatic hyperplasia. J Urol. 2005;173:1256.
4. Ziada A, Rosenblum M, Crawford E. Benign prostatic hyperplasia: an overview. J Urol. 1999;53:1–6.
5. Eckhardt M, Van Venrooij G, Boon T. Symptoms, prostate volume, and urodynamic findings in elderly male volunteers without and with LUTS and in patients with LUTS suggestive of benign prostatic hyperplasia. Urology. 2001;58:966–71.
6. Michel M, Heemann U, Schumacher H. Association of hypertension with symptoms of benign prostatic hyperplasia. J Urol. 2004;172:1390–3.
7. Miano R, De Nunzio C, Tubaro A. Treatment of benign hyperplasia in the geriatric patient. Eur Urol Rev. 2009;4(1):15–9.
8. Kohler-Ockmore J, Feneley R. Long-term catheterization of the bladder: prevalence and morbidity. J Urol. 1996;77:347–51.
9. Armitage J, Rashidian A. The thermo-expandable metallic stent for managing benign prostatic hyperplasia: a systematic review. BJU Int. 2006;98:806–10.
10. Hoffmann R, Monga M, Elliot S. Microwave thermotherapy for benign prostatic hyperplasia (Review). Cochrane Database Syst Rev. 2012;(9):CD004135.
11. Reich O, Gratzke C. Morbidity, mortality and early outcome of transurethral resection of the prostate: a prospective multicenter evaluation of 10,654 patients. J Urol. 2008;180:246–9.
12a. Ahyai SA, Gilling P, et al. Meta-analysis of functional outcomes and complications following transurethral procedures for lower urinary tract symptoms resulting from benign prostatic enlargement. Eur Urol. 2010;58(3):384–97.
12. Reich O, Bachmann A. High power (80 W) potassium-titanyl-phosphate laser vaporization of the prostate in 66 high risk patients. J Urol. 2005;173:158–60.
13. Chung D, Wysock J. Outcomes and complications after 532 nm laser prostatectomy in anticoagulated patients with benign prostatic hyperplasia. J Urol. 2011;186:977–81.
14. Elmansy H, Baazeem A. Holmium laser enucleation versus photoselective vaporization for prostatic adenoma greater than 60 Ml: preliminary results of a prospective. Randomized Clinical Trial. J Urol. 2012;188:216–21.
15. Tyson M, Lerner L. Safety of holmium laser enucleation of the prostate in anticoagulated patients. J Endourol. 2009;23:1343–6.
16. Rigg JR, Jamrozik K, Myles PS, Silbert B, Peyton P, Parsons RW, Collins K. Design of the multicenter Australian study of epidural anesthesia and analgesia in major surgery: the master trial. Control Clin Trials. 2000;21(3):244–56.
17. Winge K, Skau A, Stimpel H. Prevalence of bladder dysfunction in Parkinsons disease. Neurourol Urodyn. 2006;25:116.
18. Fowler C. Update on the neurology of Parkinson's disease. Neurourol Urodyn. 2007;26:103.
19. Fowler C, Griffiths D, De Groat W. The neural control of micturition. Nat Rev Neurosci. 2008;9:453.
20. Wringe K, Friberg L, Werdelin L. Relationship between nigrostriatal dopaminergic degeneration, urinary tract symptoms and bladder control in Parkinson's disease. Eur J Neurol. 2005;12:842.
21. Araki I, Kuno S. Assessment of voiding dysfunction in Parkinson's disease by the international prostate symptom score. J Neurol Neurosurg Psychiatry. 2000;68:429.
22. Sakakibara R, Tateno F. Pathophysiology of bladder dysfunction in Parkinson's disease. Neurobiol Dis. 2012;46:565–71.
23. Christmas T, Kempster P, Chapple C. Role of subcutaneous apomorphine in parkinsonian voiding dysfunction. Lancet. 1988;2:1451.

24. Araki I, Kitahara M, Oida T. Voiding dysfunction and Parkinson's disease: urodynamic abnormalities and urinary symptoms. J Urol. 2000;164:1640.
25. Roth B, Studer U, Fowler C. Benign prostatic obstruction and Parkinson's disease-should transurethral resection of the prostate be avoided? J Urol. 2009;181:2209–13.
26. Aranda B, Cramer P. Effects of apomorphine and L-dopa on the parkinsonian bladder. Neurourol Urodyn. 1993;12:203.
27. Fitzmaurice H, Fowler C, Rickards D. Micturition disturbance in Parkinson's disease. Neurourol Urodyn. 1985;57:652.
28. Uchiyama T, Sakakibara R, Hattori T. Short-term effect of a single levodopa dose on micturition disturbance in Parkinson's disease. Mov Disord. 2003;18:573.
29. Giannantoni A, Conte A. Botulinum toxin type A in patients with Parkinson's disease and refractory overactive bladder. J Urol. 2011;186:960–4.
30. Staskin D, Vardi Y, Siroky M. Post-prostatectomy continence in the parkinsonian patient: the significance of poor voluntary control. J Urol. 1988;140:117.
31. Wenning G, Geser F, Stampfer K. Multiple system atrophy: an update. Mov Disord. 2003;18:34.
32. Paviour D, Williams D, Fowler C. Is sphincter electromyography a helpful investigation in the diagnosis of multiple system atrophy? A retrospective study with pathological diagnosis. Mov Disord. 2005;20:1425.
33. Wyndaele J, Castro D, Madersbacher H. Neurogenic and faecal incontinence. Incontinence. 2005;2:1059–162.
34. Nitti V. Pressure flow urodynamic studies: the gold standard for diagnosing bladder outlet obstruction. Rev Urol. 2005;7:14–21.
35. Abrams P, Bruskewitz R, De La Rosette JJ, et al. The diagnosis of bladder outlet obstruction: Urodynamics. In: Cockett ATK, Khoury S, Aso Y, et al., editors. Proceedings of the 3rd International Consultation on Benign Prostatic Hyperplasia (BPH). Chapter 7. Jersey: Scientific Communications, International Ltd; 1996. p. 297–367.
36. Abrams P, Griffiths D. The assessment of prostatic obstruction from urodynamic measurement and from residual volume. J Urol. 1979;51:129–34.
37. Dubey A, Kumar A. Acute urinary retention: defining the need and timing for pressure-flow studies. BJU Int. 2001;88:178–82.
38. Griebling T. Sacral nerve stimulation in the elderly. Int Urogynecol J. 2010;21(2):458–89.
39. Blatt A, Brammah S. Transurethral prostate resection in patients with hypocontractile detrusor-what is the predictive value of ultrastructural detrusor changes? J Urol. 2012;188:2294–9.
40. Elbadawi A, Yalla S. Structural basis of geriatric voiding dysfunction. IV Bladder outlet obstruction. J Urol. 1993;150:1681.
41. Oelke M, Höfner K. Diagnostic accuracy of noninvasive tests to evaluate bladder outlet obstruction in men: detrusor wall thickness, uroflowmetry, postvoid residual urine, and prostate volume. Eur Urol. 2007;52:827–34.
42. Huang T, Qi J. Predictive value of resistive index, detrusor wall thickness and ultrasound estimated bladder weight regarding the outcome after transurethral prostatectomy for patients with lower urinary tract symptoms suggestive of benign prostatic obstruction. J Urol. 2012;165:2010–2.
43. Ou R, Pan C. Urodynamically diagnosed detrusor hypocontractility: should transurethral resection of the prostate be contraindicated? Int Urol Nephrol. 2012;44:35–9.
44. Ghalayini I, Al-Ghazo M. A prospective randomized trial comparing transurethral prostatic resection and clean intermittent self-catheterization in men with chronic urinary retention. BJU Int. 2005;96:93–7.
45. Van Kerrebroeck E. Results of sacral neuromodulation therapy for urinary voiding dysfunction: outcomes of a prospective. Worldwide Clinical Study. J Urol. 2007;178:2029–34.
46. Emberton D, Black N. The effect of prostatectomy on symptom severity and quality of life. BJU Int. 1996;77:233–47.

47. Machino R, Kakizaki H. Detrusor instability with equivocal obstruction: A predictor of unfavorable symptomatic outcomes after transurethral prostatectomy. Neurourol Urodyn. 2002;21:444–9.
48. Zhang P, Gao J. Urodynamic analysis of non-improvement after prostatectomy. Chin Med J (Engl). 2002;115:1093–5.
49. Kuo H. Analysis of the pathophysiology of lower urinary tract symptoms in patients after prostatectomy. J Urol. 2002;68:99–104.
50. Elshal A, Hazem M. Feasibility of holmium laser enucleation of the prostate (HoLEP) for recurrent/residual benign prostatic hyperplasia (BPH). BJU Int. 2012;110:845–50.
51. Price D, Ramsden P. The unstable bladder and prostatectomy. Br J Urol. 1980;52:529–31.
52. Abrams P. The results of prostatectomy: a symptomatic and urodynamic analysis of 152 patients. J Urol. 1979;121:640–2.
53. Van Venrooji G. Correlations of urodynamic changes with changes in symptoms and well-being after transurethral resection of the prostate. J Urol. 2002;168:605–9.
54. Irwin D. Population-based survey of urinary incontinence, overactive bladder, and other lower urinary tract symptoms in five countries: results of the EPIC study. Eur Urol. 2006;50:1306–41.
55. Nitti V. OnabotulinumtoxinA for the treatment of patients with overactive bladder and urinary incontinence: results of a phase 3 R placebo-controlled trial. J Urol. 2012. doi:10.1016/j.juro.2012.12.022.

Index

A

Acute urinary retention (AUR), 62, 73, 74, 76
Alfuzosin, 69, 72
Algorithm, LUTS
   American Urological Association Guideline, 60–61
   Canadian Urology Association (2010) Guidelines, 58–60
   European Association of Urology Guidelines, 56–57
   International Consultation on Urological Diseases (2006), 61
   NICE Guidelines, 57–58
   South African Urological Association Guideline (2006), 61–62
Alpha-blockers
   conservative, LUTS, 57, 60
   first-line drug therapy, 61
American Urological Association (AUA) Guidelines
   conservative and drug treatment, 60–61
   surgery, 61
5α-reductase inhibitors (5-ARIs)
   Alfuzosin-Finasteride study, 72
   AUR/BPH, 74
   Combination of Avodart and Tamsulosin (CombAT) trial, 73–74
   dutasteride, 71
   Enlarged Prostate International Comparator (EPIC) study, 72
   finasteride inhibits, 71
   LUTS, 75
   MTOPS study, 72–73
   NICE guidelines, 75
   Veterans Affairs Cooperative Benign Prostatic Hyperplasia Study, 72

5-ARIs. *See* 5α-reductase inhibitors (5-ARIs)
AUR. *See* Acute urinary retention (AUR)

B

Benign prostatic enlargement (BPE), 15–16
Benign prostatic hyperplasia (BPH)
   American Urological Association Guideline, management, 60–61
   BOO and DO, 154–155
   Canadian Urology Association (2010) Guidelines, 58–60
   histological diagnosis, 21
   laparoscopic adenomectomy, 129–133
   management, patients, 47–48
   pathological, 22
   pressure–flow studies, 45
   progression, 39, 40
   and prostate cancer concern, 60
   RASP (*see* Robotic-assisted simple prostatectomy (RASP))
   single-site surgery, 139–140
   South African Urological Association Guideline (2006), 61–62
   TEAP, 141–142
   urethral lift, 140–141
Benign prostatic obstruction (BPO)
   prostatectomy (*see* Simple prostatectomy)
   recommendations, surgery, 90
   TUERP and TURisV, 101
Bladder outlet obstruction (BOO)
   DWT, 153
   OAB, 155
   secondary surgery, 155
   TURP, 154
   urinary retention, 153
   uroflowmetry, 152

Bladder wall thickness (BWT), 43–44
α-Blockers, 69–71
BOO. *See* Bladder outlet obstruction (BOO)
BPE. *See* Benign prostatic enlargement (BPE)
BPH. *See* Benign prostatic hyperplasia (BPH)
BPO. *See* Benign prostatic obstruction (BPO)
BWT. *See* Bladder wall thickness (BWT)

C
Canadian Urology Association (2010) Guidelines
  BPH and prostate cancer concern, 60
  BPH-related bleeding, 60
  lifestyle modifications, 58–59
  monopolar TURP, 59–60
  optional medical treatment, 59
  symptomatic prostatic enlargement, 60
Cardiovascular diseases (CVD)
  a1-AR antagonists, 147
  anticoagulant therapy, 149
  HoLEP, 148–149
  KTP laser vaporization, 148
  life expectancy, 146–147
  LMWH, 149
  patients' characteristics, 150
  spinal anesthesia *vs.* general anesthesia, 149
  TUMT and TUNA, 147–148
  urethral/suprapubic catheterization, 147
Chronic urinary retention (CUR)
  catheterization, 63, 64
  International Continence Society, 62
  NICE definition, 63
CISC. *See* Clean intermittent self-catheterization (CISC)
Clean intermittent self-catheterization (CISC), 63, 154, 155
Clinical practice guidelines (CPGs), 34
Comorbidities
  cardiovascular (CV), 146–150
  neurogenic, 150–154
Conservative, LUTS
  alpha-blocker, 57, 60
  5-ARIs, 60–61
  treatment of men, storage LUTS, 58, 59
  urethral milking, 57
CUR. *See* Chronic urinary retention (CUR)
CVD. *See* Cardiovascular diseases (CVD)

D
The Danish Prostate Symptom Score (DAN-PSS), 37
DAN-PSS. *See* The Danish Prostate Symptom Score (DAN-PSS)

Detrusor failure (DF)
  BOO (*see* Bladder outlet obstruction (BOO))
  CISC and TURP, 154
  clinical sign, 152
  DWT and UEBW, 153
  UD diagnosis, 152
  ultrastructural analysis, 153
  urinary retention, 153
Detrusor overactivity (DO)
  apomorphine, 150
  cystometry and pressure-flow study, 152
  OAB, 155
Detrusor wall thickness (DWT), 43, 153, 154
DF. *See* Detrusor failure (DF)
Diagnosis, LUTS/BPO
  blood tests, 38–39
  endoscopy, lower urinary tract, 46
  frequency–volume charts, 39–40
  imaging
    bladder and detrusor wall thickness, 43–44
    urinary tract ultrasound, 42
  PVR urine, 40–41
  recommendations, 35
  urinalysis, 38
  urodynamics, 44–46
  uroflowmetry, 41
DiLEP. *See* Diode laser enucleation of the prostate (DiLEP)
Diode laser enucleation of the prostate (DiLEP), 122–123
Diode laser vaporization of the prostate (DLVP), 122–123
Disease management
  algorithms, 46–49
  EAU guidelines, 49
  European Association of Urology guidelines, LUTS, 49
  NICE guidelines, 49–50
  patients with LUTS, 47, 48
  6th International Consultation on New Developments in Prostate Cancer and Prostatic Diseases, 46–48
DLVP. *See* Diode laser vaporization of the prostate (DLVP)
DO. *See* Detrusor overactivity (DO)
Dutasteride, 71, 72, 74
DWT. *See* Detrusor wall thickness (DWT)

E
Endoscopy, lower urinary tract, 46
Enlarged prostate gland (EPG), 15
EPG. *See* Enlarged prostate gland (EPG)
Epidemiology, BPH and LUTS

Index

economic impact, 23–24
prevalence
　detrimental effects, 23
　International Prostatic Symptom
　　Score (IPSS), 22
　maximum urinary flow rate, 23
　pathological, 22
　pelvic magnetic resonance imaging, 23
European Association of Urology (EAU)
　Guidelines, 34, 56–57

F
Finasteride, 71–73
Frequency-volume charts (FVC), 39–40
FVC. *See* Frequency-volume charts (FVC)

H
History of urology
　benign prostatic hyperplasia, 2–4
　conservative treatment, 11–13
　LUTS, 14–17
　male genitalia, anterior view, 3
　operative procedures, 9
　perineal prostatectomy
　　partial prostatectomies, 9
　　postoperative complications, 10
　　visualized extraurethral technique, 10
　prostate, 2
　prostatism, 14
　retropubic prostatectomy, 11, 13
　"Retropubic Urinary Surgery", 12
　suprapubic prostatectomy, 10–11
　transurethral procedures
　　catheterisation, 4–5
　　catheters, 6
　　Davis-Bovie generator, 7, 8
　　high-frequency unipolar current, 6
　　hollow cane-shafts, 6
　　microchip cameras, 8
　　radiotherm, 7
　　resectoscope, 7
　　Stern-McCarthy prostatic resectoscope, 7, 9
　　transurethral prostatectomy, 8
　　urethroscopic median bar excisor, 6
　treatment concept, 13–14
HoLEP. *See* Holmium laser enucleation of the prostate (HoLEP)
Holmium laser enucleation of the prostate (HoLEP), 148–150, 155
Holmium laser resection of the prostate (HoLRP)
　description, 108
　drawbacks and complications, 117–118
　equipment
　　end-fire laser fiber, 108, 111
　　transurethral resection system, 108
　intra-and postoperative complication rate, 114–115
　laser prostatectomy techniques, 113, 115
　LUTS treatment, 113–114
　physical characteristics, 116
　RCTs, 115
　rigorous prostate cancer screening, 116
　surgical technique
　　after morcellation, 113
　　incisions, 111, 112
　　modified upside-down enucleation, 113, 114
　　our lateral mobilization, side lobes, 113, 114
　　sucking, tissue, 112
　TURP, 116
HoLRP. *See* Holmium laser resection of the prostate (HoLRP)

I
ICS. *See* International Continence Society (ICS)
ICUD. *See* International Consultation on Urological Diseases (ICUD)
The International Consultation on Incontinence Questionnaire: ICIQ-Male LUTS, 37
International Consultation on Urological Diseases (ICUD), 37, 61
International Continence Society (ICS), 15, 37
International Prostatic Symptom Score (IPSS), 36
IPSS. *See* International Prostatic Symptom Score (IPSS)

K
Kalium-titanyl-phosphate (KTP), 148, 150
KTP. *See* Kalium-titanyl-phosphate (KTP)

L
Laparo-endoscopic single-site (LESS) surgery, 139
Laparoscopic adenomectomy, BPH
　advantages, 132
　bladder catheter, 131
　bladder stones, 131
　description, 129–130
　extraperitoneal transvesical approach, 132

Laparoscopic adenomectomy, BPH (cont.)
  finger-assisted technique, 132
  Hasson trocar, 130
  hemostasis, 131
  intraoperative complications, 132–133
  vs. open surgery, 133, 135
  pneumoextraperitoneum, 130
  preparation, 130
  Q_{max} and I-PSS values, 133, 134
  reepithelialization, 131
  urinary tract infections, 133
  Veress needle, 130
Laser techniques
  DiLEP and DLVP, 122–123
  diode lasers, 122
  PVP/HoLEP, 109, 110, 122
  Tm:YAG, 122
LESS surgery See Laparo-endoscopic single-site (LESS) surgery
LHRH. See Luteinizing hormone-releasing hormone (LHRH)
LMWH. See Low-molecular-weight heparin (LMWH)
Lower urinary tract symptoms (LUTS)
  aging population, 145–146
  bladder outflow obstruction, 14–15
  BPH in men, 15
  conservation (see Conservative, LUTS)
  CVD (see Cardiovascular diseases (CVD))
  DF, 152–154
  DLVP and DiLEP, 122–123
  emptying/ voiding symptoms, 16
  epidemiology (see Epidemiology, BPH and LUTS)
  and erectile dysfunction (ED), 118
  expression, 16
  filling/storage symptoms, 16
  history and physical examination, 34–36
  HoLEP, 113–114
  multifactorial aetiology, 17
  pathophysiology (see Pathophysiology)
  PD, 150–152
  post-micturition symptoms, 16
  primary care management, guideline, 62
  storage symptoms, 15
  sugical treatment (see Surgical treatment, LUTS)
  treatment algorithms (see Algorithm, LUTS)
  urinalysis and biochemical testing, 38–39
  voiding symptoms, 15

Low-molecular-weight heparin (LMWH), 149
Luteinizing hormone-releasing hormone (LHRH), 82
LUTS. See Lower urinary tract symptoms (LUTS)

M
Medical Therapy of Prostatic Symptoms (MTOPS) study, 38–39, 72–73
Medical treatment
  anticholinergic drugs, 75–77
  5-ARIs (see 5α-reductase inhibitors (5-ARIs))
  α-blockers, 69–71
  botulinum toxins, 80
  ED and ejaculatory dysfunction, 83
  LHRH, 82
  mirabegron, 81–82
  nonsurgical, 68–69
  NX-1207, 82
  onabotulinumtoxinA, 81
  PDE5-Is, 78–80
  phytotherapy, 77–78
Midstream specimen of urine (MSU), 38
MSA. See Multiple system atrophy (MSA)
MSU. See Midstream specimen of urine (MSU)
MTOPS study See Medical Therapy of Prostatic Symptoms (MTOPS) study
Multiple system atrophy (MSA), 151
Mushroom technique, 117

N
National Institute for Health and Clinical Excellence (NICE) Guidelines
  conservative and drug treatment, 57
  CUR definition, 63
  surgery, 57–58
National Overactive Bladder Evaluation (NOBLE), 37–38
Neodymium–yttrium–aluminum–garnet (Nd:YAG) laser, 118–119
NICE. See National Institute for Health and Clinical Excellence (NICE)
NOBLE. See National Overactive Bladder Evaluation (NOBLE)
Nocturia and Nocturnal Polyuria
  antimuscarinic therapy, 65
  causes, 63
  frequency-volume chart, 63–65
  treatment, 65

Index

O
OAB. *See* Overactive bladder (OAB)
OAB-Q. *See* The Overactive Bladder Questionnaire (OAB-Q)
Overactive bladder (OAB), 150–151, 155
The Overactive Bladder Questionnaire (OAB-Q), 37–38

P
Parkinson's disease (PD)
   apomorphine, 150
   botulinum toxin type A, 151
   cystometry and pressure-flow study, 152
   DO (*see* Detrusor overactivity (DO))
   neurodegeneration, 150
   OAB, 150–151
   prevalence, 150
   symptoms, 151
   TURP and MSA, 151
Pathophysiology
   etiology
      androgen-dependent tissue, 25
      apoptotic index, 25
      5α-reductase, 25
      chronic inflammation, 25–26
      dihydrotestosterone (DHT), 25
      estrogens role, 25
      local hypoxia, 26
      metabolic syndrome, 26, 27
      pro-inflammatory cytokines, upregulation, 26
      prostatic cells, abnormal proliferation, 26
      TGF-β regulates proliferation, 25
      tissue-remodeling process, 24–25
   natural history, 28
   pathogenesis
      abnormal collagen production and detrusor instability, 27
      autonomic nervous system over-activity, 27
      periurethral and transitional zone nodules, 26
      prostatic smooth muscle tone, 27
PD. *See* Parkinson's disease (PD)
PDE5-Is. *See* Phosphodiesterase type 5 inhibitors (PDE5-Is)
Perineal prostatectomy, 9–10
PFS. *See* Pressure-flow study (PFS)
Phosphodiesterase type 5 inhibitors (PDE5-Is), 78–80
Photoselective vaporization of the prostate (PVP)
   description, 118–119
   drawbacks and complications, 121
   equipment, 119
   indications and outcomes, 120–121
   surgical technique, 119–120
Phytotherapy, 77–78
Post-void residual (PVR) urine, evaluation, 40–41
Potassium titanyl phosphate (KTP) laser, 118, 119
Pressure-flow study (PFS), 44–45
Prostate, digital rectal examination, 35–36
Prostate-specific antigen (PSA), 39
Prostatism, 14
PSA. *See* Prostate-specific antigen (PSA)
PVP. *See* Photoselective vaporization of the prostate (PVP)

R
Randomized clinical trials (RCTs)
   comparing TUIP and TURP, 101
   laser techniques, TURP/OP, 109–110
   open prostatectomy *vs.* TURP, 94
   photoselective vaporization, 99
   PVP, 120
RASP. *See* Robotic-assisted simple prostatectomy (RASP)
RCTs *See* Randomized clinical trials (RCTs)
Retention
   acute urinary retention, 62
   chronic urinary retention, 62–63
Retropubic prostatectomy, 11
Risk factors, 24
Robotic-assisted simple prostatectomy (RASP)
   advantages, 137
   bladder neck, 136
   data, 137, 138
   description, 133
   finger-assisted technique, 137
   horizontal cystotomy incision, 136
   mean operation time, 136
   modifications, 136–137
   open adenomectomy, 137
   retropubic space, Retzius, 136

S
Side-firing technique, 119
Silodosin, 70, 71

Simple prostatectomy
  complications and a durable success, 92, 93
  guidelines, 95, 96
  hemostatic sutures, 91
  perineal prostatectomy, 91
  puboprostatic ligaments, 92
  retropubic technique, 91–92
  suprapubic approach, 90
  TURP (*see* Transurethral resection of the prostate (TURP))
Suprapubic prostatectomy, 10–11
Surgical treatment, LUTS
  BPO, methods, 56–57
  HoLRP (*see* Holmium laser resection of the prostate (HoLRP))
  laser techniques, 122–123
  open prostatectomy, 61
  PVP, 118–122
  TUMT and TUNA, 61

T
Tadalafil, 79–80
Tamsulosin, 70, 76–78
TEAP. *See* Transurethral ethanol ablation of the prostate (TEAP)
Thulium laser, 122, 123
Thulium–yttrium–aluminum–garnet (Tm:YAG) laser, 122
Transurethral enucleation and resection of the prostate (TUERP), 101
Transurethral ethanol ablation of the prostate (TEAP), 141–142
Transurethral incision of prostate (TUIP), 42, 96, 100–101
Transurethral microwave therapy (TUMT), 147–149
Transurethral needle ablation (TUNA), 42, 147–149
Transurethral resection of the prostate (TURP)
  bipolar electrosurgical technology, 97
  blood transfusion, 99–100
  blood transfusions, 148
  CISC, 154
  dorsal lithotomy position, 91
  electrophysiological principles, 98
  and HoLEP, 99
  long-term outcomes, 95, 97
  monopolar, 95
  morbidity, 95
  MSA, 151
  nationwide analysis, 100
  photoselective vaporization, 99
  RCTs study, 98–99
  vs. treatment options, 97, 98
  UEBW, 153
TUERP. *See* Transurethral enucleation and resection of the prostate (TUERP)
TUIP. *See* Transurethral incision of prostate (TUIP)
TUMT. *See* Transurethral microwave therapy (TUMT)
TUNA. *See* Transurethral needle ablation (TUNA)
TURP. *See* Transurethral resection of the prostate (TURP)

U
UEBW. *See* Ultrasound-estimated bladder weight (UEBW)
Ultrasound-estimated bladder weight (UEBW), 153
Urethral milking, 57
Urethrocystoscopy. *See* Endoscopy, lower urinary tract
Urinalysis, 38
Urodynamics, 44–46
Uroflowmetry, 41
UroLift, 140–141

V
Visual laser ablation of the prostate (VLAP), 118
VLAP. *See* Visual laser ablation of the prostate (VLAP)

The manufacturer's authorised representative in the EU is Springer Nature Customer Service Centre GmbH, Europaplatz 3, 69115 Heidelberg, Germany. If you have any concerns regarding our products, please contact ProductSafety@springernature.com

Printed and bound by CPI Group (UK) Ltd, Croydon, CR0 4YY

23/03/2026

02076369-0008